DR. BARBARA'S NATURAL HEALING SECRETS

The Lost Guide to Barbara O'Neill's Teachings on Herbal Remedies and Natural Healing for Holistic Health

Hannah Dawson

Table of Contents

PREFACE

Prepare to unlock a vault of hidden knowledge and discover a treasure trove of secrets curated and preserved by Dr. Barbara O'Neill, a revered sage in the realm of natural healing. As you turn the pages of this book, you will initiate yourself into a world where ancient wisdom revitalizes modern life, offering each reader keys to deeper health and profound well-being.

Dr. Barbara's teachings, once accessible only to her inner circle of students, are now available to you through this comprehensive guide. These teachings offer a robust alternative to the conventional health narratives that dominate our society today. With each chapter, you are invited to journey beyond the boundaries of traditional medicine, exploring potent herbal remedies that rejuvenate the body, holistic dietary practices that restore balance, and lifestyle adjustments that not only prevent but heal diseases.

This book serves as your personal guide through the intricacies of Dr. Barbara's methods and the deep-rooted philosophy that underpins them. Her approach is the result of a lifetime of research, practice, and a profound respect for the natural world. As you delve deeper, you will encounter the core principles of her teachings, which integrate seamlessly with actionable steps to transform your health and life.

As you embark on this path, you will find that this journey challenges you to reconsider what you thought you knew about health. You are encouraged to question the practices that have become standard yet remain unfulfilling, and to rethink the quick fixes that promise much but deliver little.

In your hands, you hold not just a collection of health tips but a manifesto of healing wisdom passed down through generations, now distilled into practical, accessible knowledge that can change lives. This book invites you to step into a space of learning and growth, where the secrets of natural healing are revealed through a tapestry of personal anecdotes, scientific research, and transformative insights.

Your journey through these pages will be one of discovery and revelation. You will uncover the hidden mechanisms of your body's own healing capabilities, learn how to harness the power of the earth's bounty, and understand how simple, everyday choices can lead to extraordinary changes in your health and vitality.

Prepare to challenge your assumptions, to embrace new ways of living and being healthy. Prepare to be transformed, for within these pages lie not only Dr. Barbara's secrets but also the path to your own personal renaissance in health.

Embark on this journey with an open heart and a curious mind. The secrets within are powerful and transformative—true keys to longevity and vitality. Welcome to your healing journey; let the revelations and transformations begin.

INTRODUCTION: A JOURNEY INTO HOLISTIC HEALTH

Embark on a transformative exploration into holistic health, guided by the enlightened teachings of Dr. Barbara O'Neill. Her profound insights and age-old practices open a gateway to a deeper understanding of wellness that transcends the superficial layers of health tips and tricks. This journey is an invitation to dive deep into a lifestyle where the delicate balance of body, mind, and spirit forms the bedrock of true wellness. Within these pages, the venerable wisdom of natural healing intertwines seamlessly with cutting-edge insights, crafting a sustainable approach to health that resonates through every aspect of life.

Imagine walking through a lush garden, where every leaf and bloom offers a story of healing and harmony—this is the essence of Dr. Barbara's world. Her holistic approach is like a tapestry woven from vibrant threads of nutrition, herbal medicine, and conscious lifestyle choices, each strand representing a vital component of health. This philosophy not only challenges but also enriches conventional medical wisdom, offering a refreshing contrast to the often mechanical and impersonal nature of modern healthcare.

As you turn each page, you will journey through Dr. Barbara's foundational teachings, which are not just lessons but life experiences shared from her heart. You will hear stories of those who have walked this path before you, like Sarah, a middle-aged woman whose battle with chronic fatigue seemed endless until she embraced the holistic practices discussed in this book. Through simple yet profound changes in her diet and daily routine, she rediscovered vitality—a testament to the power of holistic healing.

Or consider Mark, who suffered from severe digestive issues that no medication could alleviate. It was only when he turned to the herbal remedies and nutritional wisdom that Dr. Barbara champions that he began to see a world free from pain and discomfort. His journey is a beacon for all who seek relief and a peaceful coexistence with their bodies.

This book is structured to build upon itself, each chapter a stepping stone to greater understanding and health. As you immerse yourself in Dr. Barbara's teachings, you will learn how to harness the natural rhythms of your body, how to use herbal concoctions to enhance your health, and how to make lifestyle choices that promote longevity and happiness. Each lesson is designed to help you live more fully, turning everyday decisions into opportunities for wellness and joy.

This journey into holistic health is not a quick fix but a profound transformation. It will change how you view health, influencing not only the choices you make but also the very essence of how you live. Prepare to open your mind and heart to a new way of thinking about your body and your health.

Discovering the Path to Natural Wellness

Understanding and interpreting the subtle signals your body sends is a critical component of holistic health. Each sensation, whether a fleeting discomfort or a persistent pain, acts as a communication from your body about its internal conditions. This deep awareness encourages a proactive approach to health, moving beyond merely reacting to symptoms to embracing a comprehensive strategy that addresses the root causes of health issues.

This holistic approach involves a thorough understanding of how various lifestyle factors—diet, stress, sleep patterns, and physical activity—interact with personal health. By focusing on these foundational aspects, you cultivate an environment conducive to overall well-being. Rather than resorting to quick pharmaceutical fixes that may only mask symptoms, the emphasis is on natural remedies and health practices that support the body's inherent healing capabilities.

Herbal remedies are integral to this process. These natural treatments provide gentle yet powerful means to adjust bodily functions and restore balance. From soothing teas to healing tinctures, herbs like chamomile for relaxation, ginger for digestion, or turmeric for inflammation are used not just for their symptomatic relief but for their holistic benefits that contribute to long-term health.

Nutritional strategies are equally crucial. What you eat can profoundly impact your health, influencing everything from immune function to energy levels. This approach doesn't just skim the surface with generic diet plans but delves into how specific foods can be used therapeutically. For instance, incorporating anti-inflammatory foods such as leafy greens and omega-3 rich fish can help combat chronic inflammation, a root cause of many diseases. Similarly, antioxidant-rich berries and nuts can enhance cellular health and longevity.

Mindful practices such as meditation, yoga, and deep breathing complement the physical aspects of natural wellness. These techniques help to harmonize the mind and body, reducing stress and enhancing overall mindfulness, which has been linked to significant improvements in various physical health indicators, including enhanced immune function, better digestion, and reduced risk of heart disease. Engaging regularly in these practices builds resilience and promotes a balanced internal state, facilitating a natural flow of energy and vitality.

By integrating these elements into daily life, individuals not only take charge of their health in the present but also lay a robust foundation for future well-being. This proactive stance not only helps to prevent diseases but also empowers individuals to lead vibrant, energetic lives. This holistic path is not just about avoiding illness but about optimizing each aspect of life, ensuring that vitality and wellness are continually renewed and preserved.

CHAPTER 1
THE PILLARS OF HOLISTIC HEALTH

Exploring the Foundations of a Life Well-Lived

Holistic health, an ancient yet perpetually relevant concept, stands firmly on the pillars that support a life of comprehensive well-being. These pillars—physical health, mental clarity, emotional balance, and spiritual fulfillment—are not independent entities but interwoven aspects of a full and vibrant life. Understanding and nurturing each of these aspects is crucial for anyone seeking to live not just longer, but better.

Physical Health: The Foundation of Vitality

Physical health is perhaps the most visible pillar of holistic health. It involves nurturing the body through nutrition, exercise, and sleep. Proper nutrition is fundamental, fueling the body with the necessary nutrients to function optimally, fight off diseases, and repair itself. Exercise, too, plays a critical role, not only in maintaining physical fitness and bodily functions but also in boosting mood and cognitive function through the release of endorphins. Additionally, restorative sleep is essential for physical health, as it allows the body to repair itself and consolidate memories, supporting both physical and mental health.

Mental Clarity: Enhancing Cognitive Function

Mental clarity is achieved through practices that foster focus, creativity, and cognitive flexibility. Engaging in activities that challenge the mind, such as puzzles, reading, and learning new skills, can enhance mental agility and delay cognitive decline. Furthermore, mindfulness practices like meditation can improve concentration, reduce stress, and contribute to a greater sense of control over one's thoughts and emotions, leading to clearer thinking and better decision-making.

Emotional Balance: Cultivating Emotional Intelligence

Emotional balance involves managing and understanding emotions in a way that fosters resilience, reduces stress, and promotes happiness. Techniques for achieving emotional balance include practicing mindfulness, which helps individuals observe their emotions without judgment; developing coping strategies to deal with stress; and fostering positive relationships that provide support and companionship. Additionally, engaging in activities that bring joy and satisfaction can greatly enhance emotional health, contributing to a more fulfilling life.

Spiritual Fulfillment: Connecting with Deeper Meanings

Spiritual fulfillment can mean different things to different people, but generally, it involves connecting with something larger than oneself, which can provide a sense of purpose and meaning in life. This could be through organized religion, personal spirituality, or community involvement. Practices such as prayer, meditation, or spending time in nature can also nurture the spiritual self, providing peace and perspective on life's challenges.

By building strong foundations in these four pillars, individuals can create a holistic health regimen that not only prevents diseases but also enhances their quality of life. This chapter delves deep into each pillar, offering practical advice and strategies to strengthen them, thereby paving the way for a life well-lived, marked by vitality, clarity, balance, and fulfillment. This holistic approach to health is not merely about extending life but enriching its every moment.

Unlocking Your Body's Silent Language

The human body is a complex, finely tuned system equipped with an incredible capacity to heal itself. This chapter delves into the often-overlooked language of the body, revealing how it communicates its needs and how we can listen and respond to facilitate natural healing processes. Understanding this silent language is key to unlocking our innate healing powers and fostering a deeper connection with our own health.

Recognizing the Signs and Symptoms

Every ache, pain, and irregularity has significance and is part of the body's dialogue, alerting us to imbalances and potential health issues. Learning to recognize these signs is the first step in understanding the body's language. For example, persistent headaches could indicate stress, dehydration, or the need for a vision check, while digestive disturbances might suggest dietary issues or deeper gastrointestinal problems. This section will guide you through common symptoms and their possible meanings, empowering you to make informed health decisions.

The Body's Self-Repair Mechanisms

Our bodies have built-in repair systems designed to heal wounds, fight infections, and restore balance. These systems operate without conscious input, driven by the biological imperative to maintain homeostasis. This part explores key aspects of the body's self-repair mechanisms, such as the roles of the immune system, the importance of the inflammatory response in healing, and how cellular repair processes are triggered by various signals within the body.

Enhancing Natural Healing

While the body can handle minor injuries and infections on its own, there are ways to enhance its natural healing abilities. This includes optimal nutrition that provides the necessary building blocks for repair, adequate hydration to keep cellular processes running smoothly, and sufficient sleep which is crucial for recovery and regeneration. Additionally, managing stress is vital as chronic stress can suppress the immune response and slow down healing. Practical tips and lifestyle adjustments that bolster the body's healing powers will be provided, making it easier to support your body's health naturally.

Listening to Your Body Through Mindfulness

Mindfulness and meditation can significantly enhance your ability to interpret your body's signals. By fostering a heightened awareness of bodily sensations and emotional states, mindfulness practices help you tune into subtle signs that might otherwise go unnoticed. This section includes exercises designed to improve body awareness, such as guided meditations and mindfulness routines that can be incorporated into daily life, enhancing your capacity to listen to and understand your body's needs.

Integrating Body Intelligence into Daily Life

Finally, integrating the knowledge of the body's language into everyday life is crucial for long-term health maintenance. This means making lifestyle choices that consistently support the body's natural healing abilities and adjusting these choices as your body's needs change over time. Strategies for maintaining this integration, including regular check-ins with your body and adjustments to your health regimen, will be discussed to ensure that you remain in tune with your body's silent language as your life evolves.

By unlocking and understanding your body's silent language, you not only enhance your ability to heal naturally but also take proactive steps towards maintaining your health and preventing future illnesses. This chapter provides the tools and knowledge to navigate and harness the complexities of your body's natural healing capabilities, empowering you with the confidence to care for your well-being effectively.

CHAPTER 3
MASTERING HERBAL MEDICINE

The Art and Science of Nature's Pharmacy

Herbal medicine represents a profound synthesis of art and science, offering a time-honored approach to healing that uses the curative properties of plants. This chapter delves deep into the realm of herbalism, exploring its historical roots, scientific backing, and practical applications. By understanding how to effectively harness the power of nature's pharmacy, you can integrate herbal remedies into your health regimen to promote healing, prevent illness, and enhance overall well-being.

Historical Perspectives and Modern Validation

The use of plants for healing dates back thousands of years, forming the backbone of traditional medicine systems across the world, from Ayurveda in India to Traditional Chinese Medicine. In this section, we'll trace the origins of herbal medicine, illustrating how ancient wisdom aligns with contemporary scientific research. Modern studies increasingly validate what herbalists have known for centuries: plants contain potent compounds that can treat a wide array of health issues effectively and safely.

Active Compounds and Their Healing Properties

Plants are complex organisms that produce an array of chemical compounds; many of these, such as flavonoids, alkaloids, and terpenes, have therapeutic effects. This part of the chapter will explain how these compounds work at the molecular level to improve health, such as by reducing inflammation, combating free radicals, or modulating hormone levels. Understanding the active components of herbs is crucial for both recognizing their potential uses and appreciating the scientific foundation of herbal medicine.

Crafting Your Herbal Apothecary

Building your own herbal apothecary is both empowering and practical. This section will guide you through selecting, storing, and using a wide range of essential herbs. From the calming effects of lavender and chamomile to the digestive benefits of ginger and peppermint, you will learn how to prepare basic herbal formulations such as teas, tinctures, salves, and oils. We will also discuss proper dosage, potential side effects, and how to customize herbal treatments to individual needs.

Integrating Herbal Remedies into Daily Life

Herbal medicine isn't just for treating illness; it's also about maintaining health and wellness. This part will explore ways to incorporate herbs into daily routines for optimal health benefits. Whether it's starting the day with a tonic tea, using adaptogenic herbs to manage stress, or applying herbal ointments for skin care, you'll discover how to make herbal practices both effective and enjoyable.

Ethical and Sustainable Practices

As the popularity of herbal medicine grows, so does the need for sustainable and ethical practices in harvesting and consuming medicinal plants. This section addresses the importance of sourcing herbs responsibly to ensure that both the environment and the cultures that depend on these plants are respected and protected. We'll cover how to choose suppliers who prioritize sustainability and how you can even grow your own herbs to guarantee purity and reduce environmental impact.

Ancient Remedies for the Modern Age

Herbal medicine bridges the gap between ancient wisdom and modern health challenges. As we navigate the complexities of contemporary life, with its stress, pollution, and fast-paced demands, the gentle yet potent properties of herbs offer a soothing balm. In this age of rising chronic conditions and mental health concerns, revisiting the time-tested remedies provided by nature can be particularly effective.

The Impact of Modern Lifestyles on Health

Modern lifestyles contribute significantly to a range of health issues. Chronic stress, anxiety, and sleep disorders have become prevalent, alongside lifestyle-related diseases such as diabetes and hypertension. Environmental factors like pollution and sedentary habits compound these issues, creating a cycle of health complications that demand innovative approaches to health and wellness.

Relieving Stress and Anxiety with Herbs

Herbs such as ashwagandha, lavender, and lemon balm have long histories of calming the mind and promoting relaxation. Ashwagandha, an adaptogen, helps the body manage stress more effectively by moderating the stress response system. Lavender, often used in aromatherapy, is renowned for its ability to reduce anxiety and improve sleep quality. Lemon balm, with its mild sedative properties, can decrease anxiety and promote a sense of calm.

Herbal Approaches to Physical Health

Herbs also play a crucial role in managing and preventing physical ailments exacerbated by modern life. For instance, turmeric, with its potent anti-inflammatory properties, is effective in managing conditions like arthritis and metabolic syndrome. Ginger, another powerful herb, supports digestion and can alleviate symptoms of nausea and inflammation.

Herbs like ginseng and ginkgo biloba enhance cognitive function and energy levels, addressing the fatigue and mental fog that often plague individuals in high-stress environments. By improving circulation and boosting brain health, these herbs help maintain cognitive functions and overall vitality.

Integrating Herbal Remedies Into Daily Life

Incorporating herbal remedies into daily routines is an accessible way to enhance health naturally. Simple practices, such as starting the day with a cup of herbal tea or using herbal supplements, can make significant improvements in overall well-being. Moreover, creating personal blends of herbs for specific conditions like insomnia or indigestion personalizes the healing experience, making it more effective and enjoyable.

Herbal medicine offers a profound connection to nature and its healing capabilities. By utilizing these ancient remedies, we not only address specific health issues but also enhance our overall well-being, proving that even in our modern world, the wisdom of the past holds key solutions for today's ailments.

Food as Medicine: What Would Dr. Barbara Eat?

In this chapter, we delve into the concept of food as a fundamental tool for healing and maintaining health. Dr. Barbara advocates a diet that is not only nutritious but also medicinal, supporting the body's natural processes and helping to prevent the onset of disease. Understanding how to utilize food as medicine can transform the way we approach our daily meals and our overall health.

Principles of a Healing Diet

A healing diet emphasizes whole, nutrient-dense foods that provide a plethora of health benefits. Dr. Barbara's approach involves selecting foods that enhance digestive health, boost immune function, and stabilize energy levels throughout the day. The focus is on fresh fruits and vegetables, whole grains, lean proteins, and healthy fats, each chosen for their specific health-promoting properties.

Key Concept: Whole Foods vs. Processed Foods

- **Whole Foods:** Naturally occurring foods that are consumed in their original form, minimally processed, and devoid of added ingredients such as preservatives, artificial flavors, or colorings. They are rich in essential nutrients like vitamins, minerals, fiber, and antioxidants.

- **Processed Foods:** Foods that have been altered from their natural state, often through manufacturing processes, and typically contain additives such as sugars, oils, salts, and preservatives. These foods are generally lower in nutrients and higher in calories, which can contribute to health issues like obesity, diabetes, and heart disease.

Anti-Inflammatory Foods

Inflammation is a natural bodily response to injury and infection, but chronic inflammation can lead to numerous health problems. Incorporating anti-inflammatory foods into the diet can help mitigate this risk. Foods rich in omega-3 fatty acids, such as salmon and flaxseeds, as well as turmeric, blueberries, and leafy greens, have strong anti-inflammatory properties.

Gut Health and Its Importance

The health of the gut impacts overall health profoundly, influencing everything from immune function to mental health. A diet rich in probiotics (found in yogurt and fermented foods like kimchi and sauerkraut) and prebiotics (found in foods like onions, garlic, and bananas) supports a healthy digestive tract and a robust microbiome.

Key Concept: Probiotics vs. Prebiotics

- **Probiotics:** Live beneficial bacteria that are ingested through foods or supplements, which add to the population of good bacteria in the digestive system.

- **Prebiotics:** Non-digestible food components (mainly fibers) that promote the growth of beneficial bacteria in the gut by serving as food for them.

Balancing Macronutrients

Balancing macronutrients (carbohydrates, proteins, and fats) is essential for optimizing health. Dr. Barbara emphasizes the importance of selecting high-quality sources of each:

- **Carbohydrates:** Opt for whole grains, legumes, and starchy vegetables to provide energy and fiber.

- **Proteins:** Include lean meats, fish, eggs, and plant-based proteins such as lentils and chickpeas to support tissue repair and muscle growth.

- **Fats:** Focus on unsaturated fats found in nuts, seeds, avocados, and olive oil, which support heart health and cellular function.

Seasonal and Local Eating

Eating according to the seasons and choosing local foods not only supports local economies but also provides you with the freshest and most nutrient-dense produce. Seasonal foods are harvested at their peak and are typically richer in vitamins and minerals than out-of-season counterparts that have traveled long distances.

A Treasure Trove of Healing

In this chapter, we explore 25 herbal remedies that, although less common, hold significant medicinal properties according to the teachings of Dr. Barbara. These herbs, often overlooked in mainstream herbal medicine, are prized in various traditional practices for their unique healing abilities. Here's a list of these valuable herbs, each chosen for its potential to contribute to overall health and well-being:

Astragalus Tea Recipe

Benefits: Astragalus is renowned for its ability to boost the immune system and combat fatigue. This simple tea recipe is an easy way to incorporate astragalus into your daily routine to help enhance vitality and overall health.

Ingredients:

- 1-2 tablespoons of dried astragalus root slices

- 1 liter of water

- Honey or lemon (optional, for taste)

Preparation:

1. Boil Water: Start by bringing the water to a boil in a medium-sized pot.

2. Add Astragalus: Add the dried astragalus root slices to the boiling water.

3. Simmer: Reduce the heat and let the mixture simmer gently for about 30 to 45 minutes. The longer you allow the astragalus to simmer, the stronger the tea will be.

4. Strain: Remove the pot from the heat and strain the tea into a cup or a teapot, discarding the astragalus slices.

5. Flavor: If desired, add honey or a squeeze of lemon to enhance the flavor.

6. Serve: Enjoy this tea warm. For best results, drink 1-2 cups daily, especially during times when you need an immune boost or feel more fatigued than usual.

Tips:

- Storage: You can make a larger batch and store it in the refrigerator for up to three days. Warm it slightly before drinking.

- Combination: Astragalus pairs well with other immune-boosting herbs like ginger or ginseng. Consider adding a small piece of fresh ginger while simmering to enhance the tea's flavor and benefits.

This astragalus tea serves as a simple yet effective way to harness the herb's health-promoting properties, offering a natural boost to your immune system and energy levels.

Bupleurum Liver Support Tea Recipe

Benefits: Bupleurum is a staple in Traditional Chinese Medicine, often used to enhance liver function and establish emotional balance. This herbal tea blend combines bupleurum with other supportive herbs to create a therapeutic drink that nurtures the liver and soothes the mind.

Ingredients:

- 1 teaspoon of dried bupleurum root
- 1 teaspoon of dried peppermint leaves
- 1/2 teaspoon of dried licorice root
- 1/2 teaspoon of dried dandelion root
- 4 cups of water

Preparation:

1. Boil Water: Bring water to a boil in a medium-sized pot.

2. Add Herbs: Once the water is boiling, add the bupleurum, peppermint, licorice, and dandelion roots to the pot.

3. Simmer: Reduce the heat and allow the mixture to simmer for about 15-20 minutes. The

simmering helps extract the full range of active compounds from the herbs.

4. Strain: After simmering, remove the pot from the heat and strain the mixture into a large mug or teapot, discarding the spent herbs.

5. Serve: Drink this tea warm. You can enjoy it up to twice a day, especially during periods when you feel your liver might be stressed or when experiencing emotional upheaval.

Tips:

- Flavor Adjustments: If the taste is too bitter due to the dandelion and licorice, you can adjust the amount of peppermint or add a bit of honey to sweeten it naturally.

- Usage: This tea is particularly beneficial during times of dietary excess or when you are feeling sluggish, both physically and emotionally.

- Precautions: Bupleurum can interact with certain medications and is not recommended for pregnant or breastfeeding women. As with any herbal treatment, consult with a healthcare provider before starting a new regimen, especially if you have existing health conditions or are taking other medications.

This Bupleurum Liver Support Tea is a thoughtful way to integrate the benefits of traditional Chinese herbs into your daily health routine, supporting your liver function and contributing to emotional stability.

Codonopsis Energy Boost Tonic Recipe

Benefits: Codonopsis is often hailed as a milder alternative to ginseng, making it ideal for those who might find ginseng too stimulating. This tonic is designed to enhance energy and vitality without over-stimulating the body, providing a sustainable boost that supports overall well-being.

Ingredients:

- 1 tablespoon of dried Codonopsis root

- 1 tablespoon of goji berries

- 1 small slice of fresh ginger

- 1 cinnamon stick

- 4 cups of water

Preparation:

1. Boil Water: Bring the water to a boil in a saucepan.

2. Add Ingredients: Once boiling, add the Codonopsis root, goji berries, ginger slice, and cinnamon stick to the water.

3. Simmer: Reduce the heat to low and allow the mixture to simmer gently for about 30 minutes. This slow simmering helps to extract the beneficial properties of the ingredients effectively.

4. Strain: After simmering, take the saucepan off the heat and strain the liquid into a large mug or heatproof container, removing all solid pieces.

5. Serve: Enjoy this tonic warm. For an added touch of sweetness and to enhance the flavor, a teaspoon of honey can be stirred into the warm tonic before drinking.

Tips:

- Daily Use: This tonic can be consumed daily, ideally in the morning, to help kickstart your day with enhanced energy.

- Storage: If you make a larger batch, you can store the strained tonic in the refrigerator for up to 3 days. Gently reheat before consuming.

- Enhancements: For additional benefits, consider adding a small piece of licorice root to the simmering process, which can help support adrenal function and further improve energy levels.

This Codonopsis Energy Boost Tonic leverages the gentle, yet effective, energy-enhancing properties of Codonopsis, combined with other synergistic ingredients, to provide a balanced boost that revitalizes both body and mind. It's an excellent choice for anyone looking to increase their vitality naturally without the intense effects of stronger stimulants like traditional ginseng.

Rhodiola Rosea Energy Elixir Recipe

Benefits: Rhodiola Rosea is celebrated for its ability to enhance mental clarity and physical endurance, making it an excellent herb for those who need a boost in cognitive and physical performance. This elixir combines Rhodiola with complementary ingredients that support sustained energy and focus.

Ingredients:

- 1 teaspoon of Rhodiola Rosea powder
- 1 cup of hot water (not boiling, as too high heat can destroy some active compounds)
- 1 teaspoon of raw honey (optional, for taste)
- A squeeze of fresh lemon juice (to enhance absorption of active compounds)
- A pinch of cinnamon (for flavor and additional cognitive benefits)

Preparation:

1. Prepare Water: Heat water until it is hot but not boiling. About 185°F (85°C) is ideal, as it extracts the herb's properties effectively without degrading them.
2. Mix Ingredients: Place the Rhodiola Rosea powder in a mug. Add the hot water to the mug, stirring well to ensure the powder is fully dissolved.
3. Add Flavors: Stir in the raw honey, fresh lemon juice, and a pinch of cinnamon. Mix thoroughly until all components are well blended.
4. Let It Steep: Allow the mixture to steep for about 10 minutes. This steeping time lets the flavors meld and ensures maximum extraction of Rhodiola's beneficial properties.
5. Serve: Once steeped, stir again and enjoy the elixir warm.

Tips:

- Consumption Time: It's best to consume this elixir in the morning or early afternoon to make the most of its energizing effects without interfering with nighttime sleep.
- Storage: This drink is best enjoyed fresh, but if you need to make it ahead of time, it can be stored in the refrigerator for up to 24 hours. Give it a good stir before drinking, as the powder might settle.
- Variations: For a cooling summer drink, prepare the elixir in advance and chill it in the refrigerator. Serve over ice for a refreshing and invigorating beverage.

This Rhodiola Rosea Energy Elixir is designed to provide a natural uplift to both your mental and physical states, helping to improve focus, reduce mental fatigue, and increase stamina. It's a simple yet potent way to incorporate the adaptogenic benefits of Rhodiola into your daily routine.

Benefits: Schisandra berries are renowned for their adaptogenic properties, which make them an excellent choice for promoting liver health and aiding in stress relief. This tea recipe harnesses the full potential of Schisandra berries to enhance your body's resilience to stress and support liver function.

Ingredients:

- 2 teaspoons of dried Schisandra berries
- 1 liter of water
- 1 teaspoon of honey (optional, to sweeten)
- A slice of lemon (optional, for added flavor and vitamin C)

Preparation:

1. Boil Water: Bring the water to a boil in a medium-sized pot.
2. Add Schisandra Berries: Once the water is boiling, add the dried Schisandra berries. Reduce the heat to a simmer.
3. Simmer: Let the berries simmer gently for about 20-30 minutes. The longer you simmer, the more intense the flavor and the extraction of beneficial compounds.
4. Strain: Remove the pot from the heat and strain the liquid, removing the berries. Press the berries gently to extract maximum juice and beneficial properties.
5. Enhance Flavor: Add a teaspoon of honey and a slice of lemon to the warm tea for flavor enhancement. Stir well to dissolve the honey.
6. Serve: Enjoy this tea warm or let it cool and drink it as a refreshing cold beverage.

Tips:

- Frequency and Timing: Drinking a cup of Schisandra berry tea twice daily can significantly support liver health and stress management. It's particularly beneficial to drink this tea in the morning to jump-start liver function and late in the afternoon to combat end-of-day fatigue.
- Storage: You can store any extra tea in the refrigerator for up to 48 hours. Reheat gently or enjoy chilled, as preferred.

- Additional Uses: Schisandra berries can also be incorporated into various dishes, such as cereals, smoothies, and yogurts, to take advantage of their health benefits in different forms.

This Schisandra Berry Liver Detox Tea is a powerful tool in your wellness regimen, offering a natural method to support liver health and relieve stress. The adaptogenic qualities of Schisandra help balance the body's stress response while actively promoting overall vitality and wellness.

Eucommia Bone and Joint Health Tonic Recipe

Benefits: Eucommia is highly valued for its ability to support bone health, enhance joint mobility, and promote cardiovascular health. This tonic combines Eucommia with other supportive ingredients to create a potent drink that aids in strengthening the body's structural systems and supporting heart health.

Ingredients:

- 1 tablespoon of dried Eucommia bark

- 1 liter of water

- 1 teaspoon of turmeric powder (for anti-inflammatory properties)

- A small piece of ginger root, thinly sliced (for additional anti-inflammatory and cardiovascular benefits)

- Honey to taste (optional, for sweetness)

Preparation:

1. Boil Water: Bring the water to a boil in a medium saucepan.

2. Add Ingredients: Once boiling, reduce the heat to a simmer and add the dried Eucommia bark, turmeric powder, and slices of ginger root to the water.

3. Simmer: Allow the mixture to simmer gently for about 20-30 minutes. This slow cooking process helps to extract the active compounds from the Eucommia bark effectively.

4. Strain: Remove the saucepan from the heat and strain the tonic through a fine mesh sieve into a large jug or container, discarding the solids.

5. Sweeten: If desired, stir in honey while the tonic is still warm to enhance the flavor.

6. Serve: This tonic can be consumed warm or chilled. For best results, drink one cup of the tonic daily, especially during times of increased physical activity or when you feel your joints and bones need extra support.

Tips:

- Storage: If you have leftover tonic, it can be stored in the refrigerator for up to 3 days. Make sure to stir well before serving, as some sediments might settle at the bottom.

- Variations: For those who prefer a more robust flavor, add a cinnamon stick during the simmering process for its warming qualities and additional circulatory benefits.

- Additional Benefits: Regular consumption of this Eucommia tonic can help reduce general inflammation, support joint lubrication, and enhance overall mobility, making it especially beneficial for those with joint discomfort or those at risk for bone density issues.

This Eucommia Bone and Joint Health Tonic is an excellent way to harness the therapeutic properties of Eucommia, ginger, and turmeric in a simple, everyday beverage. Its natural compounds are specifically beneficial for maintaining bone density, improving joint function, and supporting cardiovascular health, making it a vital addition to a holistic health regimen.

He Shou Wu Rejuvenating Elixir Recipe

Benefits: He Shou Wu, also known as Fo-Ti, is celebrated in traditional herbal medicine for its rejuvenating and toning properties. This elixir is designed to tap into the root's potential to enhance vitality, improve hair health, and boost longevity.

Ingredients:

- 1 tablespoon of dried He Shou Wu (Fo-Ti) root

- 1 liter of water

- 1 tablespoon of goji berries (for additional antioxidant benefits)

- A few slices of fresh orange (for flavor and vitamin C)

- Honey to taste (optional, for sweetness)

Preparation:

1. Prepare He Shou Wu: Pre-soak the dried He Shou Wu root in cold water for an hour before boiling. This helps to remove any impurities and enhances the extraction of beneficial compounds.

2. Boil Water: After soaking, drain the He Shou Wu root and add it along with 1 liter of fresh water to a saucepan. Bring it to a boil.

3. Add Ingredients: Once the water is boiling, reduce the heat to a simmer. Add the goji berries and fresh orange slices to the pot.

4. Simmer: Let the mixture simmer gently for 30 to 40 minutes. The longer simmer time allows thorough extraction of the He Shou Wu's rejuvenating properties.

5. Strain and Sweeten: Remove from heat, strain the elixir into a heat-resistant container, and discard the solids. If desired, add honey while the elixir is still warm to sweeten.

6. Serve: Enjoy this elixir warm, or let it cool down and drink it chilled for a refreshing tonic. It can be consumed daily, preferably in the morning, to capitalize on its revitalizing effects throughout the day.

Tips:

- Regular Use: For best results, integrate this elixir into your daily routine for extended periods. He Shou Wu is known for its cumulative benefits, improving with regular use.

- Storage: This elixir can be stored in the refrigerator for up to 48 hours. Ensure to stir or shake well before consuming if settled.

- Enhancements: To further boost its health benefits, consider adding a slice of ginger or a pinch of cinnamon during the simmering process. These spices will enhance the elixir's warming properties and increase its circulatory benefits.

This He Shou Wu Rejuvenating Elixir recipe provides a potent way to enjoy the health benefits of this traditional herb, along with the added nutritional advantages of goji berries and oranges. Regular consumption can help improve overall vitality, strengthen hair and nails, and support a healthy aging process.

Baikal Skullcap Respiratory Relief Tea Recipe

Benefits: Baikal Skullcap is a powerful herb traditionally used in herbal medicine to treat respiratory infections and reduce inflammation. This tea recipe harnesses the therapeutic properties of Baikal

Skullcap to provide respiratory support and help alleviate symptoms associated with colds, flu, and other respiratory ailments.

Ingredients:

- 1 teaspoon of dried Baikal Skullcap root
- 1 liter of water
- 1 teaspoon of dried peppermint leaves (to enhance respiratory benefits and add flavor)
- 1 teaspoon of honey (optional, for sweetness and soothing properties)
- A slice of lemon (for vitamin C and to enhance flavor)

Preparation:

1. Boil Water: Bring the water to a boil in a medium saucepan.
2. Add Skullcap and Peppermint: Once the water reaches a boil, add the Baikal Skullcap root and dried peppermint leaves.
3. Simmer: Turn down the heat and let the mixture simmer gently for about 15-20 minutes. This duration allows for the extraction of the active compounds from the herbs.
4. Strain: After simmering, remove the saucepan from the heat. Strain the tea into a large mug or a teapot, removing all solid materials.
5. Add Lemon and Honey: Stir in a slice of lemon and a teaspoon of honey while the tea is still warm. The lemon adds a refreshing zest and vitamin C, which is crucial for immune support, while the honey provides a soothing effect and natural sweetness.
6. Serve: Drink this tea warm, ideally during or just before the onset of respiratory symptoms. It can be consumed 2-3 times a day when fighting an infection.

Tips:

- Enhancing the Blend: For an extra immune boost, consider adding a small piece of ginger or a few cloves of garlic to the brew. Both are known for their antimicrobial and anti-inflammatory properties.
- Storage: If you prepare a larger batch, the tea can be stored in the refrigerator for up to 48 hours. Reheat gently before drinking.
- Usage Considerations: Baikal Skullcap is potent and should be used with caution. It's advisable

to consult with a healthcare provider before starting any new herbal treatment, especially for those on medication or with pre-existing health conditions.

This Baikal Skullcap Respiratory Relief Tea is a practical and natural way to utilize the benefits of this traditional herb to support respiratory health. Regular consumption can help manage symptoms during respiratory infections and contribute to overall lung and immune health.

Rehmannia Menstrual and Kidney Health Tonic Recipe

Benefits: Rehmannia is revered in traditional medicine for its effectiveness in regulating menstrual cycles and supporting kidney health. This tonic leverages these properties to provide relief from menstrual discomfort and enhance kidney function.

Ingredients:

- 1 tablespoon of dried Rehmannia root

- 1 liter of water

- 1 teaspoon of cinnamon powder (for blood sugar regulation and added flavor)

- 1 tablespoon of cranberry juice (for kidney health and urinary tract support)

- Honey to taste (optional, for sweetness)

Preparation:

1. Boil Water: Bring the water to a boil in a medium saucepan.

2. Add Rehmannia: Add the dried Rehmannia root to the boiling water.

3. Simmer: Reduce the heat and allow the mixture to simmer for about 30 minutes to fully extract the root's beneficial properties.

4. Add Cinnamon: Stir in the cinnamon powder during the last 5 minutes of simmering.

5. Strain and Flavor: Remove from heat, strain out the solids, and add the cranberry juice. Sweeten with honey if desired.

6. Serve: Drink this tonic warm, ideally 1-2 cups daily, starting a few days before and continuing through the menstrual period for best results in regulating the cycle.

Spilanthes Antimicrobial Immune Boosting Tonic Recipe

Benefits: Known for its potent antibacterial and immune-stimulating properties, Spilanthes is an effective herb for boosting the immune system and combating bacterial infections.

Ingredients:

- 1 teaspoon of dried Spilanthes flowers and leaves

- 1 liter of water

- Juice of 1 lemon (for immune support and flavor)

- Honey to taste (optional, for sweetness)

Preparation:

1. Boil Water: Bring the water to a boil in a large pot.

2. Add Spilanthes: Once boiling, add the Spilanthes flowers and leaves.

3. Simmer: Reduce the heat and simmer for about 15 minutes.

4. Strain and Enhance: Strain the liquid, then add fresh lemon juice. Sweeten with honey if preferred.

5. Serve: Consume this tonic warm to maximize benefits, especially during the cold and flu season or when feeling susceptible to infections.

White Willow Bark Natural Pain Relief Tea

Benefits: White Willow Bark has been used as a natural precursor to aspirin for pain relief. This tea is especially effective for reducing headaches, back pain, and other inflammatory-related discomfort.

Ingredients:

- 2 teaspoons of dried White Willow Bark

- 1 liter of water

- 1 teaspoon of dried peppermint leaves (for flavor and digestive benefits)

- Honey to taste (optional, for sweetness)

Preparation:

1. Boil Water: Bring the water to a boil in a saucepan.

2. Add Willow Bark and Peppermint: Add White Willow Bark and peppermint leaves to the boiling water.

3. Simmer: Let the mixture simmer for about 20 minutes; this allows the salicin from White Willow Bark to be released.

4. Strain: Remove from heat and strain the tea into a mug.

5. Sweeten: Add honey if needed for sweetness.

6. Serve: Drink this tea warm, ideally when experiencing pain to take advantage of its anti-inflammatory properties.

Wild Yam Digestive and Women's Health Tea

Benefits: Wild Yam is renowned for its supportive role in women's health and its effectiveness in easing digestive issues. This tea combines the root's properties to promote hormonal balance and improve digestive functions.

Ingredients:

- 1 tablespoon of dried Wild Yam root

- 1 liter of water

- 1 teaspoon of ginger (optional, for additional digestive benefits)

- Honey (optional, for sweetness)

Preparation:

Boil 1 liter of water in a saucepan and add 1 tablespoon of dried Wild Yam root. Allow it to simmer for about 20 minutes to effectively extract the active compounds. After simmering, strain the liquid into a cup and add a teaspoon of freshly grated ginger for enhanced digestive benefits and flavor. If preferred, sweeten with honey. This tea is best enjoyed twice daily, particularly beneficial for women experiencing menopausal symptoms or menstrual discomfort.

Black Cohosh Menopause Relief Tonic

Benefits: Black Cohosh is extensively used to manage menopause symptoms and menstrual pain, providing natural relief from hot flashes, night sweats, and mood swings.

Ingredients:

- 1 teaspoon of dried Black Cohosh root

- 1 liter of water

- Lemon slices (for flavor)

- Honey (optional, for sweetness)

Preparation:

Start by boiling 1 liter of water in a pot. Add 1 teaspoon of dried Black Cohosh root and reduce heat, allowing it to simmer gently for 15-20 minutes. This will help release the beneficial properties of the herb. Strain the mixture into a mug, add a few slices of lemon for a refreshing taste, and sweeten with honey if desired. Drink this tonic once daily to alleviate menopause symptoms and ease menstrual pain.

Mullein Respiratory Soothing Tea

Benefits: Mullein is excellent for treating respiratory conditions, helping to clear congestion and soothe irritated mucous membranes.

Ingredients:

- 2 teaspoons of dried Mullein leaves

- 1 liter of water

- Honey (optional, for soothing effect and sweetness)

Preparation:

Bring 1 liter of water to a boil and add 2 teaspoons of dried Mullein leaves. Simmer on low heat for about 15 minutes to allow the leaves to infuse their medicinal properties into the water. Strain the tea into a large mug and add honey to enhance the soothing effect and flavor, especially beneficial when dealing with a cough or respiratory irritation. Consume this tea several times a day when experiencing respiratory discomfort.

Boswellia Joint Health Tea

Benefits: Boswellia is celebrated for its anti-inflammatory properties, especially effective in enhancing joint health and relieving pain.

Ingredients:

- 1 teaspoon of Boswellia resin

- 1 liter of water

- A pinch of ground turmeric (for additional anti-inflammatory benefits)

- Honey (optional, for sweetness)

Preparation:

In a saucepan, bring 1 liter of water to a boil and add 1 teaspoon of Boswellia resin. Simmer for 20 minutes to extract the active compounds. To boost its anti-inflammatory effects, add a pinch of ground turmeric towards the end of simmering. Strain and sweeten with honey if desired. Drink this tea regularly to support joint health and reduce inflammation.

Hawthorn Berry Cardiovascular Tea

Benefits: Hawthorn Berry is known to promote cardiovascular health and regulate blood pressure.

Ingredients:

- 2 teaspoons of dried Hawthorn berries

- 1 liter of water

- Honey (optional, for sweetness)

Preparation:

Boil 1 liter of water and add 2 teaspoons of dried Hawthorn berries. Let it simmer for 20 minutes to allow the berries to release their beneficial properties fully. Strain the mixture into a mug and, if desired, sweeten with honey. Drinking this tea daily can help maintain a healthy cardiovascular system and manage blood pressure levels.

Ashoka Tonic for Women's Health

Benefits: Ashoka is a revered herb in Ayurvedic medicine, particularly known for its benefits in enhancing female reproductive health, including regulating menstrual cycles and relieving pain associated with conditions like endometriosis.

Ingredients:

- 1 tablespoon of dried Ashoka bark
- 1 liter of water
- 1 teaspoon of fennel seeds (for additional hormone balancing effects)
- Honey (optional, for sweetness)

Preparation:

In a pot, bring 1 liter of water to a boil and add the dried Ashoka bark along with fennel seeds. Reduce the heat and simmer for 30 minutes to allow the herbs to release their potent properties into the water. Strain the mixture and add honey to sweeten if desired. Drink this tonic daily to help regulate menstrual cycles and support overall uterine health.

Gotu Kola Brain Tonic

Benefits: Gotu Kola is known for its ability to enhance cognitive function and support circulatory health, making it ideal for boosting brain activity and improving blood flow.

Ingredients:

- 1 teaspoon of dried Gotu Kola leaves
- 1 liter of water
- Lemon zest (for a refreshing flavor)
- Honey (optional, for sweetness)

Preparation:

Bring 1 liter of water to a boil and add the dried Gotu Kola leaves. Simmer on low heat for 20 minutes to infuse the water with the herb's cognitive-enhancing properties. Add lemon zest in the last few minutes for a refreshing taste. Strain the tea, add honey if desired, and drink it once or twice daily to enhance mental clarity and memory retention.

Andrographis Cold and Flu Remedy

Benefits: Andrographis is highly effective in treating the symptoms of colds and flu, as well as reducing inflammation, making it a go-to remedy during the flu season.

Ingredients:

- 1 teaspoon of dried Andrographis leaves

- 1 liter of water

- A few slices of fresh ginger (for added immune support)

- Honey (optional, for sweetness)

Preparation:

Boil 1 liter of water and add dried Andrographis leaves and slices of fresh ginger. Reduce the heat and let it simmer for 15 minutes. The combination works synergistically to boost the immune system and alleviate flu symptoms. Strain and sweeten with honey to make the remedy more palatable. Consume this drink at the first sign of cold or flu symptoms up to three times a day.

Bacopa Monnieri Stress Relief Tea

Benefits: Bacopa Monnieri is traditionally used to enhance memory and reduce stress, supporting overall brain health and reducing anxiety.

Ingredients:

- 1 teaspoon of dried Bacopa Monnieri leaves

- 1 liter of water

- A pinch of cinnamon (for flavor and additional cognitive benefits)

- Honey (optional, for sweetness)

Preparation:

Bring 1 liter of water to a boil and then add the dried Bacopa Monnieri leaves. Include a pinch of cinnamon for flavor and added cognitive benefits. Let the mixture simmer for 20 minutes to fully extract the herb's stress-relieving properties. Strain the tea into a cup, add honey if desired, and drink once daily to enjoy enhanced memory function and reduced mental stress.

Neem Detox Tea

Benefits: Neem is renowned for its anti-parasitic and detoxifying properties, making it an excellent choice for cleansing the body and supporting immune health.

Ingredients:

- 1 teaspoon of dried Neem leaves

- 1 liter of water

- A few mint leaves (to improve taste and add digestive benefits)

- Lemon slices (for detoxifying vitamin C and flavor)

Preparation:

Begin by boiling 1 liter of water in a saucepan. Add the dried Neem leaves and reduce the heat to let it simmer for about 15 minutes. Neem can be quite bitter, so adding a few fresh mint leaves and lemon slices towards the end of the simmering process can help mitigate the bitterness and enhance the flavor. Strain the tea into a cup or pitcher, and consume this detox tea once daily, preferably in the morning, to take advantage of its cleansing effects on the body.

Guggul Metabolism Boosting Tea

Benefits: Guggul is well-regarded for its ability to manage cholesterol levels and enhance metabolism, contributing to cardiovascular health and weight management.

Ingredients:

- 1 teaspoon of Guggul resin

- 1 liter of water

- Half a cinnamon stick (for additional metabolic support and flavor)

- Honey (optional, for sweetness)

Preparation:

Boil 1 liter of water and add the Guggul resin along with half a cinnamon stick to enhance the metabolic effects and provide a pleasant flavor to the tea. Allow the mixture to simmer for about 20 minutes, letting the active compounds fully infuse the water. Strain the tea, add honey if desired for sweetness, and drink once daily to support metabolism and cholesterol management.

Shatavari Women's Health Elixir

Benefits: Shatavari is considered a crucial herb for women, traditionally used to support fertility, hormonal balance, and overall vitality.

Ingredients:

- 1 tablespoon of dried Shatavari root

- 1 liter of water

- A few slices of ginger (to enhance absorption and add warmth)

- Honey (optional, for sweetness)

Preparation:

Heat 1 liter of water to a boil and add the dried Shatavari root along with a few slices of ginger, which can help with absorption and add a warming effect. Simmer the mixture for approximately 25 minutes to extract the full benefits of the herb. Strain the elixir and sweeten with honey if desired. Drink this elixir daily, particularly beneficial for women seeking to enhance reproductive health and hormonal balance.

Licorice Root Digestive Soothing Tea

Benefits: Licorice Root is famous for its ability to soothe gastrointestinal problems and restore balance to the digestive system.

Ingredients:

- 1 teaspoon of dried Licorice Root
- 1 liter of water
- A pinch of fennel seeds (to enhance digestive benefits and flavor)
- Honey (optional, for sweetness)

Preparation:

Bring 1 liter of water to a boil and add the dried Licorice Root and a pinch of fennel seeds, which complement the digestive benefits of Licorice and improve the tea's flavor profile. Reduce heat and simmer for about 15 minutes. Strain the mixture into a mug, sweeten with honey if preferred, and consume this tea up to twice daily to help soothe the digestive system and promote gastrointestinal health.

Castor Oil: Dr. Barbara O'Neill's Secret to Holistic Healing

Benefits: Castor oil, a cornerstone of Dr. Barbara O'Neill's healing arsenal, is celebrated for its remarkable anti-inflammatory, antibacterial, and laxative properties. It is a versatile oil, used both topically and internally to treat a wide array of health conditions from skin ailments and pain relief to enhancing digestive wellness. This section explores the profound uses of castor oil, revealing why it is considered one of the hidden gems in the world of natural healing.

The Healing Powers of Castor Oil

Castor oil is derived from the seeds of the Castor plant (Ricinus communis), and its healing powers have been documented for thousands of years across various cultures. Its main component, ricinoleic acid, is what gives castor oil its powerful therapeutic properties. When used topically, castor oil penetrates deeply into the skin, promoting blood circulation, relieving pain, reducing inflammation, and enhancing the healing of tissues. Internally, it acts as a stimulant laxative, providing relief from constipation and cleansing the digestive system by inducing bowel movements.

Topical Applications: Pain Relief and Skin Health

Pain Relief Compress: Castor oil compresses are an effective remedy for reducing pain and inflammation. Soak a piece of wool flannel in castor oil, place it on the affected area (such as joints, muscles, or the abdomen), cover with plastic wrap, and apply a heating pad. The heat helps the oil penetrate deeper into the tissues, providing relief from pain, inflammation, and even detoxifying internal organs when applied to the abdomen.

Skin Health: Castor oil is a natural moisturizer rich in fatty acids, which can enhance skin health by promoting hydration, elasticity, and a clear complexion. It can be applied directly to dry patches, scars, or stretched skin to improve moisture content and promote healing. Its antibacterial properties also make it beneficial for treating acne-prone skin by fighting bacteria that can cause breakouts.

Internal Use: Digestive Cleanser

Digestive Health: For constipation relief, Dr. Barbara recommends a small dose of castor oil taken internally. The recommended approach is to take 1-2 teaspoons of castor oil in the morning on an empty stomach. The oil works as a stimulant laxative, quickly clearing the intestines and colon, which can detoxify the body and help restore regular bowel movements. This should not be a regular practice but used occasionally when experiencing severe constipation or detoxification.

Safety and Precautions

While castor oil is incredibly beneficial, it should be used with caution. When applying topically, always do a patch test first to ensure there is no allergic reaction. Pregnant women should avoid using castor oil, especially internally, as it can induce labor. For internal use, it is crucial not to overuse castor oil due to its potent laxative effects, which can lead to dehydration and electrolyte imbalances if not managed carefully.

Dr. Barbara's Insider Tips

To fully harness the potential of castor oil, Dr. Barbara suggests integrating it into regular wellness routines cautiously and judiciously. For persistent issues, whether digestive, inflammatory, or skin-related, incorporating castor oil treatments over several weeks can yield profound healing benefits. Always source cold-pressed, pure, hexane-free castor oil to ensure the best quality for health use.

Incorporating castor oil into your health regimen, as advised by Dr. Barbara O'Neill, can be a powerful way to enhance well-being naturally. Whether used as a compress for pain, a skin treatment, or a digestive aid, castor oil's versatile and potent properties make it a must-have in the natural health toolkit.

Benefits: This special recipe for a Castor Oil Pack harnesses the therapeutic properties of castor oil in a method that maximizes its anti-inflammatory, detoxifying, and pain-relieving potential. This technique is particularly effective for abdominal complaints, liver detoxification, menstrual pain, and inflammation reduction.

Ingredients:

- High-quality, cold-pressed, hexane-free castor oil

- Cotton or wool flannel large enough to cover the affected area

- Plastic wrap or a plastic bag

- A heating pad or hot water bottle

- Old clothes and towels (castor oil can stain)

Preparation and Application:

1. Prepare the Area: Choose a comfortable place where you can lie down and relax. It's important to wear old clothes and use old towels, as castor oil can stain fabric permanently.

2. Soak the Flannel: Pour enough castor oil onto the flannel to saturate it, but not so much that it is dripping. The flannel should be wet but not overly soaked. You might need to fold the flannel to fit the size of the area you are treating.

3. Apply to the Body: Place the saturated flannel over the target area, such as the abdomen for digestive issues or the joints for pain relief. Cover the flannel with plastic wrap or a plastic bag to prevent the oil from leaking.

4. Add Heat: Place a heating pad or a hot water bottle over the plastic-covered flannel. The heat will help the castor oil penetrate deeper into the skin and increase its efficacy. Make sure the heat is comfortable and not too hot to avoid burns.

5. Relaxation Time: Lie back and relax with the pack in place for about 30-60 minutes. During this time, you can read, meditate, or simply rest. The warmth and oil work together to stimulate lymphatic circulation and soothe inflammation.

6. Cleanup: After removing the pack, cleanse the area with a solution of baking soda and water

(about a teaspoon of baking soda to a pint of water) to remove any residual oil. Wash the flannel in hot water and soap to remove the oil before storing it for future use.

7. Frequency of Use: For best results, Dr. Barbara recommends using the castor oil pack 3-4 times a week. It is particularly beneficial to use in the evening, as the relaxing effects can help improve sleep quality.

Tips:

- Storage of Flannel: Store the saturated flannel in a plastic bag in the refrigerator. You can reuse the flannel many times, adding more oil as needed to keep it saturated.

- Enhancements: To increase the therapeutic benefits, you can add a few drops of essential oils like lavender for relaxation or ginger for enhanced circulation to the castor oil before soaking the flannel.

This special castor oil pack recipe is one of Dr. Barbara O'Neill's secrets for tapping into the natural healing properties of castor oil. It provides a deeply soothing and healing treatment that is easy to implement and can make a significant difference in managing pain, enhancing detoxification, and promoting overall health.

Cooking Up Health and Happiness

This chapter is dedicated to transforming simple ingredients into nourishing meals that not only taste delicious but also enhance your overall health and vitality. Each recipe is crafted to harness the natural benefits of whole foods, tailored to support various aspects of wellness from boosting energy to improving digestion.

Quinoa and Black Bean Salad Recipe

Benefits: This salad is a powerhouse of nutrition, combining the protein-rich quinoa with fiber-packed black beans. It's ideal for boosting energy, supporting digestive health, and maintaining blood sugar levels. Perfect for a healthy lunch or a filling side dish.

Ingredients:

- 1 cup quinoa, rinsed
- 2 cups water or vegetable broth (for cooking quinoa)
- 1 can (15 ounces) black beans, rinsed and drained
- 1 red bell pepper, finely chopped
- 1/4 cup red onion, finely chopped
- 1/2 cup fresh cilantro, chopped
- 1 avocado, diced
- 1 lime, juiced
- 2 tablespoons olive oil
- Salt and pepper to taste
- Optional: 1 teaspoon ground cumin for extra flavor

Preparation:

Cook the quinoa by bringing it with water or broth to a boil in a medium saucepan, then covering and simmering on low heat until tender and all liquid is absorbed, about 15 minutes. Allow to cool. In a large bowl, mix the cooled quinoa, black beans, red bell pepper, red onion, and cilantro. Add the diced avocado, lime juice, olive oil, salt, and pepper, tossing to combine thoroughly. If desired, sprinkle with ground cumin for added flavor. This salad can be served immediately or chilled in the refrigerator before serving to enhance the flavors.

Turmeric Ginger Tea Recipe

Benefits: Turmeric Ginger Tea is a powerful drink, rich in anti-inflammatory properties, and excellent for soothing the digestive system. It's also known for boosting immunity and reducing inflammation.

Ingredients:

- 1 teaspoon of turmeric powder
- 1 teaspoon of freshly grated ginger
- 1 tablespoon of honey (optional, for sweetness)
- Juice of half a lemon
- 1 cup of boiling water

Preparation:

Start by boiling water. In a mug, combine the turmeric powder and freshly grated ginger. Pour the boiling water over these ingredients and let steep for about 5-7 minutes. Strain the mixture to remove the solids. Stir in the honey for sweetness and add lemon juice for an extra vitamin C boost. This tea can be enjoyed warm and is perfect for cold evenings or to soothe an upset stomach.

Kale and Sweet Potato Soup Recipe

Benefits: Packed with nutrients, this soup is great for immune support. Kale provides a healthy dose of vitamins C and K, while sweet potatoes are rich in vitamin A and fiber, promoting overall health and digestive wellness.

Ingredients:

- 1 large sweet potato, peeled and cubed
- 2 cups chopped kale
- 1 onion, chopped
- 2 cloves garlic, minced
- 4 cups vegetable broth
- 1 teaspoon olive oil
- Salt and pepper to taste
- Optional: red pepper flakes for a spicy kick

Preparation:

Heat olive oil in a large pot over medium heat. Add the chopped onion and minced garlic, sautéing until the onions are translucent. Add the cubed sweet potatoes and cook for a few minutes before pouring in the vegetable broth. Bring to a boil, then reduce heat and simmer until the sweet potatoes are tender. Add the chopped kale and cook until it is wilted and bright green. Season with salt, pepper, and optional red pepper flakes. Blend the soup with an immersion blender until smooth. Serve hot, garnished with a dollop of sour cream or a sprinkle of chopped herbs for an extra layer of flavor.

Oven-Roasted Salmon with Dill Sauce Recipe

Benefits: This dish is rich in omega-3 fatty acids, crucial for heart and brain health. Omega-3s help reduce inflammation, improve cholesterol levels, and support cognitive functions.

Ingredients:

- 4 salmon fillets (about 6 ounces each)
- 2 tablespoons olive oil
- Salt and black pepper to taste
- Lemon slices for garnish

For the Dill Sauce:

- 1/2 cup Greek yogurt
- 2 tablespoons chopped fresh dill
- 1 tablespoon lemon juice
- 1 clove garlic, minced
- Salt and pepper to taste

Preparation:

Preheat your oven to 400°F (200°C). Line a baking sheet with foil and lightly grease it with olive oil. Place the salmon fillets on the sheet, skin side down, and brush them with olive oil. Season with salt and pepper. Roast in the oven for 12-15 minutes, or until the salmon is cooked through and flakes easily with a fork. While the salmon is cooking, prepare the dill sauce by mixing Greek yogurt, fresh dill, lemon juice, minced garlic, salt, and pepper in a small bowl. Serve the roasted salmon garnished with lemon slices and a generous dollop of dill sauce.

Avocado and Spinach Smoothie Recipe

Benefits: This smoothie is a powerhouse of nutrients, packed with vitamins and healthy fats that are essential for skin and hair health. The combination of avocado and spinach provides vitamins E, C, and omega-3 fatty acids, which are vital for maintaining healthy skin and luscious hair.

Ingredients:

- 1 ripe avocado, peeled and pitted
- 2 cups fresh spinach leaves
- 1 banana
- 1/2 cup Greek yogurt
- 1 cup almond milk
- 1 tablespoon honey or to taste
- Ice cubes

Preparation:

Combine the avocado, spinach, banana, Greek yogurt, almond milk, and honey in a blender. Add a handful of ice cubes. Blend on high until smooth and creamy. Adjust the sweetness with more honey if needed. Pour into glasses and serve immediately. This smoothie is perfect for a quick breakfast or a refreshing afternoon snack.

Roasted Beet and Carrot Salad Recipe

Benefits: Beets and carrots are known for their liver detoxifying and blood-purifying properties thanks to their high levels of betaine and beta-carotene, which help improve liver function and cleanse the blood.

Ingredients:

- 3 medium beets, peeled and diced
- 3 large carrots, peeled and sliced
- 2 tablespoons olive oil
- 2 tablespoons balsamic vinegar
- Salt and black pepper to taste
- 1/4 cup chopped walnuts
- 1/4 cup crumbled feta cheese
- Fresh parsley, chopped for garnish

Preparation:

Preheat your oven to 400°F (200°C). Toss the diced beets and sliced carrots with olive oil, balsamic vinegar, salt, and pepper on a baking sheet. Spread them out in an even layer. Roast in the oven for 25-30 minutes, or until the vegetables are tender and caramelized. Remove from the oven and let cool slightly. Transfer the roasted beets and carrots to a salad bowl. Add chopped walnuts and crumbled feta cheese. Toss everything together. Garnish with chopped parsley before serving. This salad can be served warm or at room temperature and is excellent for a healthy lunch or as a side dish.

Coconut Curry Lentil Stew Recipe

Benefits: This hearty stew is not only comforting but also packed with metabolism-stimulating spices like turmeric, cumin, and ginger. Lentils provide an excellent source of protein and fiber, aiding in digestion and sustained energy levels.

Ingredients:

- 1 cup dried lentils, rinsed
- 1 onion, finely chopped
- 2 cloves garlic, minced
- 1 tablespoon grated ginger
- 1 tablespoon curry powder
- 1 teaspoon turmeric
- 1/2 teaspoon cumin
- 1 can (14 oz) coconut milk
- 2 cups vegetable broth
- 1 large carrot, diced
- 1 red bell pepper, diced
- Salt and pepper to taste
- Fresh cilantro, chopped for garnish
- 1 tablespoon coconut oil

Preparation:

In a large pot, heat the coconut oil over medium heat. Add the chopped onion, garlic, and ginger, sautéing until the onions are translucent. Stir in the curry powder, turmeric, and cumin, cooking for another minute until fragrant. Add the lentils, coconut milk, vegetable broth, diced carrot, and red bell pepper. Bring to a boil, then reduce heat and simmer for about 20-25 minutes or until the lentils are tender. Season with salt and pepper. Serve hot, garnished with fresh cilantro. This stew is perfect for a chilly day, providing warmth and a boost to your metabolism.

Almond and Chia Seed Pudding Recipe

Benefits: Packed with omega-3 fatty acids from chia seeds and almonds, this pudding is a fantastic source of fiber and healthy fats, promoting digestive health and providing a long-lasting feeling of fullness.

Ingredients:

- 1/4 cup chia seeds
- 1 cup almond milk
- 1 tablespoon honey or maple syrup
- 1/2 teaspoon vanilla extract
- 2 tablespoons slivered almonds
- Fresh berries for topping

Preparation:

In a bowl, combine the chia seeds and almond milk. Stir in the honey and vanilla extract. Mix well until the chia seeds begin to swell and absorb the liquid. Cover the bowl and refrigerate for at least 4 hours, or overnight, allowing the chia seeds to form a gel-like pudding. Before serving, stir the pudding to check consistency and add more almond milk if it's too thick. Top with slivered almonds and fresh berries for added flavor and nutrients. This pudding makes a nutritious breakfast or a satisfying dessert.

Broccoli and Almond Stir-Fry Recipe

Benefits: This stir-fry is an excellent source of antioxidants and Vitamin C from broccoli, coupled with the crunch and nutritional benefits of almonds.

Ingredients:

- 2 heads of broccoli, cut into florets
- 1/2 cup whole almonds
- 2 tablespoons olive oil
- 2 cloves garlic, minced

- 1 tablespoon soy sauce

- 1 teaspoon sesame oil

- Salt and pepper to taste

Preparation:

Heat the olive oil in a large skillet or wok over medium-high heat. Add the almonds and toast them lightly for about 2 minutes. Add the minced garlic and broccoli florets, stir-frying for about 5-7 minutes or until the broccoli is tender but still crisp. Drizzle with soy sauce and sesame oil, tossing to coat all the ingredients evenly. Season with salt and pepper. Serve this vibrant broccoli and almond stir-fry hot as a side dish or incorporate it into a main meal with protein like tofu or chicken. This dish not only packs a nutritional punch but also brings a delicious crunch and flavor to your meal.

Pumpkin and Ginger Muffins Recipe

Benefits: These muffins are a great source of fiber and packed with anti-inflammatory ingredients like ginger, making them perfect for a nourishing start to the day. The addition of pumpkin not only provides a moist texture but also adds a good dose of vitamin A and fiber.

Ingredients:

- 1 1/2 cups all-purpose flour (or a gluten-free alternative)

- 1/2 cup brown sugar

- 1/4 cup white sugar

- 1 teaspoon baking powder

- 1/2 teaspoon baking soda

- 1 teaspoon ground cinnamon

- 1/4 teaspoon ground nutmeg

- 1/4 teaspoon ground ginger

- 1 cup pumpkin puree

- 1/3 cup vegetable oil

- 1 egg
- 1 teaspoon vanilla extract
- 1/4 cup crystallized ginger, finely chopped

Preparation:

Preheat your oven to 350°F (175°C) and line a muffin tin with paper liners. In a large bowl, whisk together the flour, brown sugar, white sugar, baking powder, baking soda, cinnamon, nutmeg, and ground ginger. In another bowl, mix the pumpkin puree, vegetable oil, egg, and vanilla extract until smooth. Fold the wet ingredients into the dry ingredients until just combined, then stir in the crystallized ginger. Divide the batter evenly among the muffin cups. Bake for 20-25 minutes, or until a toothpick inserted into the center of a muffin comes out clean. Let them cool before serving. Enjoy these flavorful muffins as a quick breakfast or a healthy snack.

Spicy Sweet Potato Hummus Recipe

Benefits: This vibrant twist on traditional hummus is rich in beta-carotene from sweet potatoes, which is excellent for vision and immune health. The addition of spices not only enhances flavor but also boosts metabolism.

Ingredients:

- 1 large sweet potato, peeled and cubed
- 1 can (15 oz) chickpeas, drained and rinsed
- 2 tablespoons tahini
- 2 cloves garlic, minced
- Juice of 1 lemon
- 1 teaspoon paprika
- 1/2 teaspoon cumin
- 1/4 teaspoon cayenne pepper
- Salt to taste

- Olive oil for drizzling

Preparation:

Steam or boil the sweet potato cubes until tender, about 15-20 minutes. In a food processor, combine the cooked sweet potato, chickpeas, tahini, garlic, lemon juice, paprika, cumin, and cayenne pepper. Blend until smooth, adding a little water or olive oil if needed to achieve the desired consistency. Season with salt to taste. Transfer to a serving bowl and drizzle with olive oil. Serve the hummus with fresh vegetables, pita bread, or as a flavorful spread on sandwiches.

Stuffed Bell Peppers with Quinoa and Mushrooms Recipe

Benefits: These stuffed bell peppers are a complete meal with a balance of proteins from quinoa and a variety of vitamins from mushrooms and bell peppers. This dish is filling, nutritious, and visually appealing.

Ingredients:

- 4 large bell peppers, tops cut off and seeds removed
- 1 cup quinoa, cooked
- 1 cup mushrooms, finely chopped
- 1 onion, diced
- 2 cloves garlic, minced
- 1/2 cup grated Parmesan cheese
- 1/2 cup tomato sauce
- 1 tablespoon olive oil
- Salt and pepper to taste
- Fresh parsley, chopped for garnish

Preparation:

Preheat the oven to 375°F (190°C). In a skillet, heat olive oil over medium heat. Sauté the onion and garlic until translucent, then add the mushrooms and cook until they are soft and browned. In a large bowl, mix the sautéed vegetables with cooked quinoa, Parmesan cheese, and tomato sauce.

Season the mixture with salt and pepper. Stuff the mixture into the hollowed-out bell peppers, and place them in a baking dish. Cover with foil and bake for about 30 minutes. Remove the foil and bake for an additional 10 minutes, or until the peppers are tender and the tops are lightly browned. Garnish with fresh parsley before serving. Enjoy this hearty and healthy meal that perfectly balances flavor and nutrition.

Chickpea and Spinach Curry Recipe

Benefits: This nutrient-rich curry combines the iron and protein-packed chickpeas with spinach, which is high in vitamins and minerals, offering a powerful boost to energy and overall health.

Ingredients:

- 1 can (15 oz) chickpeas, drained and rinsed
- 2 cups fresh spinach leaves
- 1 onion, finely chopped
- 2 cloves garlic, minced
- 1 tablespoon grated ginger
- 1 can (14 oz) coconut milk
- 2 tablespoons curry powder
- 1 teaspoon turmeric powder
- 1 tablespoon olive oil
- Salt and pepper to taste
- Fresh cilantro, chopped for garnish

Preparation:

Heat the olive oil in a large pan over medium heat. Sauté the onion, garlic, and ginger until the onion becomes translucent. Add the curry powder and turmeric, stirring for about a minute until the spices are fragrant. Pour in the coconut milk and bring to a simmer. Add the chickpeas and cook for about 10 minutes, allowing the flavors to meld. Stir in the spinach and cook until it wilts, about 2-3 minutes. Season with salt and pepper to taste. Serve hot, garnished with fresh cilantro. This curry is not only flavorful but also highly beneficial for iron intake and protein needs.

Oat and Banana Pancakes Recipe

Benefits: These pancakes are a heart-healthy breakfast option, made with whole grains from oats and naturally sweetened with bananas, perfect for a nutritious start to your day.

Ingredients:

- 1 cup rolled oats
- 1 ripe banana
- 2 eggs
- 1/2 cup almond milk
- 1 teaspoon vanilla extract
- 1/2 teaspoon baking powder
- 1/4 teaspoon cinnamon
- Olive or coconut oil, for cooking

Preparation:

Blend the rolled oats in a blender until they reach a flour-like consistency. Add the banana, eggs, almond milk, vanilla extract, baking powder, and cinnamon to the blender. Blend until the mixture is smooth. Heat a non-stick skillet over medium heat and add a little oil. Pour small rounds of batter onto the skillet, cooking for about 2 minutes on each side or until golden brown and cooked through. Serve these warm pancakes with a drizzle of honey or a topping of fresh fruit.

Miso Soup with Seaweed and Tofu Recipe

Benefits: This classic Japanese soup is light yet packed with essential minerals from seaweed and protein from tofu, making it an excellent choice for a nourishing and restorative meal.

Ingredients:

- 4 cups water
- 2 tablespoons miso paste
- 1 cup tofu, cubed
- 1/2 cup dried seaweed, soaked and drained
- 2 green onions, chopped
- 1 tablespoon soy sauce

Preparation:

Bring the water to a simmer in a medium pot. Reduce the heat to low and add the tofu and seaweed. Allow to simmer gently for about 5 minutes. In a small bowl, dissolve the miso paste in a little bit of the warm broth to avoid clumps. Stir the dissolved miso back into the pot, being careful not to let the soup boil as this can destroy the beneficial probiotics in miso. Add the soy sauce and green onions, stirring to combine. Serve the soup warm, perfect for an uplifting and mineral-rich meal.

Green Detox Juice Recipe

Benefits: This refreshing juice is perfect for a quick detox, featuring kale, apple, cucumber, and celery, which combine to provide vitamins, hydration, and fiber. It's excellent for flushing toxins from the body, aiding digestion, and boosting energy levels.

Ingredients:

- 2 cups kale, roughly chopped
- 1 large apple, cored and sliced
- 1 cucumber, sliced
- 3 stalks celery, chopped
- 1 lemon, juiced
- 1 inch piece of ginger, peeled

Preparation:

Wash all the vegetables and fruits thoroughly. Place kale, apple, cucumber, celery, and ginger in a juicer. Process until smooth. Stir in the lemon juice to enhance flavor and add extra vitamin C. Serve the juice immediately to enjoy its maximum nutritional benefits. This juice is not only detoxifying but also invigorating, making it a perfect drink for starting the day or as a midday pick-me-up.

Tomato and Basil Bruschetta Recipe

Benefits: This classic Italian appetizer is not only delicious but also healthy, featuring tomatoes that are rich in antioxidants and basil, which provides vitamins and anti-inflammatory properties. Combined with a drizzle of olive oil, it offers a heart-healthy dose of fats.

Ingredients:

- 4 large ripe tomatoes, diced
- 1/4 cup fresh basil leaves, chopped
- 2 cloves garlic, minced
- 1 tablespoon extra virgin olive oil
- 1 teaspoon balsamic vinegar
- Salt and freshly ground black pepper to taste
- 1 baguette, sliced and toasted

Preparation:

In a mixing bowl, combine diced tomatoes, chopped basil, minced garlic, olive oil, and balsamic vinegar. Season with salt and pepper to taste. Mix well and let the mixture sit for about 10 minutes to allow flavors to meld. Spoon the tomato mixture generously onto slices of toasted baguette. Serve immediately to enjoy the fresh and vibrant flavors. This bruschetta is perfect as a starter or a light meal, providing a delicious way to enjoy the health benefits of fresh ingredients.

Zucchini Noodles with Avocado Pesto Recipe

Benefits: This dish offers a low-carb alternative to traditional pasta, using zucchini noodles which are high in vitamins and minerals, and paired with an avocado pesto that's rich in healthy fats and fiber.

Ingredients:

- 4 medium zucchini, spiralized into noodles
- 1 ripe avocado
- 1/2 cup fresh basil leaves
- 1/4 cup pine nuts
- 2 cloves garlic
- Juice of 1 lemon
- 2 tablespoons olive oil
- Salt and pepper to taste
- Cherry tomatoes for garnish (optional)

Preparation:

For the avocado pesto, combine the ripe avocado, basil leaves, pine nuts, garlic, and lemon juice in a food processor. Blend while drizzling in the olive oil until smooth. Season the pesto with salt and pepper to taste. Toss the spiralized zucchini noodles with the avocado pesto until they are well-coated. Serve the noodles immediately, garnished with cherry tomatoes for a burst of color and freshness. This dish is wonderfully satisfying yet light, making it an excellent choice for a healthy lunch or dinner.

Cauliflower Rice Pilaf Recipe

Benefits: This cauliflower rice pilaf is a fantastic low-calorie alternative to traditional rice dishes, packed with nutrients and offering a satisfying texture and flavor without the heaviness of grains.

Ingredients:

- 1 head of cauliflower, grated or processed into rice-sized pieces

- 1 onion, finely chopped

- 2 cloves garlic, minced

- 1/2 cup carrots, finely diced

- 1/2 cup peas

- 2 tablespoons olive oil

- 1/2 teaspoon turmeric (for color and health benefits)

- Salt and pepper to taste

- Fresh parsley, chopped for garnish

Preparation:

Heat olive oil in a large skillet over medium heat. Add the chopped onion and minced garlic, sautéing until the onion is translucent. Stir in the carrots and cook for a couple of minutes before adding the cauliflower rice and peas. Sprinkle with turmeric, salt, and pepper, mixing well to combine all ingredients. Cover and let the pilaf cook for about 5-7 minutes, stirring occasionally, until the vegetables are tender and the cauliflower is slightly crispy. Serve hot, garnished with fresh parsley. This dish is perfect as a side with your favorite protein or as a light meal on its own.

Baked Apple with Cinnamon and Nuts Recipe

Benefits: Baked apples are a healthy dessert option that combines the natural sweetness of apples with the aromatic warmth of cinnamon and the crunch of nuts, providing a good source of fiber and protein.

Ingredients:

- 4 large apples, cored

- 1/4 cup walnuts, chopped

- 1/4 cup almonds, chopped

- 2 tablespoons honey or maple syrup

- 1 teaspoon cinnamon

- 1/4 teaspoon nutmeg

- Butter or coconut oil for greasing

Preparation:

Preheat your oven to 350°F (175°C). Lightly grease a baking dish with butter or coconut oil. Mix the chopped walnuts, almonds, honey or maple syrup, cinnamon, and nutmeg in a small bowl. Stuff this mixture into the hollowed-out centers of the apples. Place the stuffed apples in the prepared baking dish. Bake in the preheated oven for about 30-35 minutes or until the apples are tender and the filling is bubbly. Serve warm, perhaps with a scoop of Greek yogurt or a drizzle of extra honey for added indulgence.

Lemon Garlic Roasted Chicken Recipe

Benefits: This roasted chicken is not only rich in protein but also infused with lemon and garlic, which offer detoxifying and immune-boosting properties.

Ingredients:

- 4 chicken breasts (bone-in, skin-on)
- 4 cloves garlic, minced
- 1 lemon, juiced and zested
- 2 tablespoons olive oil
- 1 teaspoon rosemary, chopped
- Salt and pepper to taste

Preparation:

Preheat the oven to 400°F (200°C). In a small bowl, combine the olive oil, lemon juice and zest, minced garlic, chopped rosemary, salt, and pepper. Place the chicken breasts in a roasting pan and rub them all over with the lemon garlic mixture, making sure some of the marinade gets under the skin for maximum flavor. Roast the chicken in the preheated oven for about 35-40 minutes or until the chicken is golden on the outside and cooked through (internal temperature should reach 165°F or 75°C). Serve hot, garnished with additional lemon slices and a sprinkle of fresh rosemary. This dish is perfect for a wholesome family dinner, offering a delicious way to enjoy the health benefits of chicken, lemon, and garlic.

Garlic Green Beans Almondine Recipe

Benefits: This dish features green beans sautéed with garlic and almonds, making it rich in heart-healthy fats, fiber, and antioxidants. It's a delicious way to boost your intake of greens while enjoying the crunchy texture of toasted almonds.

Ingredients:

- 1 pound fresh green beans, trimmed
- 3 tablespoons olive oil
- 3 cloves garlic, minced
- 1/2 cup sliced almonds
- Salt and pepper to taste
- Lemon zest for garnish (optional)

Preparation:

Heat olive oil in a large skillet over medium heat. Add the minced garlic and sliced almonds, sautéing until the almonds are lightly toasted and the garlic is fragrant. Add the green beans to the skillet, tossing to coat with the oil, garlic, and almonds. Cook for about 7-10 minutes, or until the beans are tender but still crisp. Season with salt and pepper to taste. Garnish with lemon zest before serving to add a fresh, zesty flavor. This side dish is perfect alongside grilled meats or fish, providing a crunchy, flavorful addition to any meal.

Walnut and Berry Yogurt Parfait Recipe

Benefits: Combining yogurt with walnuts and berries creates a parfait that's not only delicious but also packed with probiotics, fiber, and antioxidants. This healthy treat supports digestive health, enhances immune function, and provides essential nutrients for overall wellness.

Ingredients:

- 1 cup Greek yogurt
- 1/2 cup fresh berries (such as strawberries, blueberries, or raspberries)
- 1/4 cup walnuts, chopped

- 2 tablespoons honey or maple syrup
- A sprinkle of cinnamon (optional)

Preparation:

In a glass or jar, layer half of the Greek yogurt followed by a layer of fresh berries and a sprinkle of chopped walnuts. Drizzle some honey or maple syrup over the top. Repeat the layers until all ingredients are used. Top with a final drizzle of honey and a sprinkle of cinnamon for extra flavor. Refrigerate for at least 30 minutes before serving to allow the flavors to meld together. This parfait makes an excellent breakfast or snack, offering a delicious and nutritious way to enjoy a mix of textures and tastes.

Watermelon and Feta Salad Recipe

Benefits: This refreshing salad combines juicy watermelon with creamy feta cheese, offering hydration, a boost of protein, and a mix of sweet and savory flavors. It's particularly good for hot weather, providing electrolytes and hydration to beat the heat.

Ingredients:

- 4 cups cubed watermelon
- 1 cup crumbled feta cheese
- 1/2 red onion, thinly sliced
- 1/4 cup fresh mint leaves, chopped
- 2 tablespoons olive oil
- Juice of 1 lime
- Salt and pepper to taste

Preparation:

In a large serving bowl, combine the cubed watermelon, crumbled feta cheese, and thinly sliced red onion. In a small bowl, whisk together the olive oil, lime juice, salt, and pepper. Pour the dressing over the watermelon mixture and gently toss to coat. Sprinkle with chopped fresh mint for a refreshing flavor contrast. Serve this salad chilled to enhance its refreshing qualities. It's perfect for summer picnics, barbecues, or as a light, hydrating meal on its own.

Benefits: Kombucha is a fermented tea known for its probiotic content, which supports gut health and enhances overall vitality. Infusing kombucha with herbs adds extra health benefits, tailoring it to specific wellness needs such as boosting immunity or reducing inflammation.

Ingredients:

- 1 gallon filtered water

- 1 cup sugar (organic cane sugar is preferred)

- 8 bags of green tea or black tea

- 2 cups of starter tea from a previous batch of kombucha or store-bought (unflavored) kombucha

- 1 SCOBY (Symbiotic Culture Of Bacteria and Yeast)

- Optional: Herbal additions such as chamomile, lavender, or ginger for flavor and health benefits

Preparation:

Begin by boiling the filtered water in a large pot. Once boiling, dissolve the sugar in the water, then add the tea bags and allow them to steep until the water has cooled to room temperature. Remove the tea bags and add the starter tea, which helps acidify the brew to protect against harmful bacteria during fermentation. Place the SCOBY in the cooled tea mixture, ensuring it's fully submerged. Cover the pot with a breathable cloth (like a coffee filter or a piece of fabric) and secure it with a rubber band. Allow the kombucha to ferment at room temperature, out of direct sunlight, for 7 to 14 days. The longer it ferments, the less sweet and more vinegary it will taste.

During the final 2-3 days of fermentation, you can add herbal flavors. For example, add a few chamomile flowers, a couple of sprigs of lavender, or slices of fresh ginger to the fermenting kombucha. This will infuse the brew with the herbs' flavors and benefits. After the fermentation period is complete, remove the SCOBY and herbal additions, and transfer the kombucha to bottles, leaving about an inch of headspace at the top to allow for carbonation. Seal the bottles and let them carbonate at room temperature for another 1 to 3 days before refrigerating.

Serve your herbal kombucha chilled. It can be enjoyed daily as a refreshing, health-promoting beverage. Each batch of kombucha can be a creative experiment with different tea bases and herbal infusions, providing delicious variety and numerous health benefits tailored to your preferences and needs.

Lifestyle Synergies

Incorporating natural healing into daily life involves creating a harmonious blend of diet, exercise, stress management, and mindfulness. Each element supports the other, enhancing overall wellness and building a foundation that naturally combats disease and promotes longevity.

Nutrition as the Cornerstone Adopting a diet rich in whole foods, fresh vegetables, fruits, whole grains, lean proteins, and healthy fats is essential. Regularly including anti-inflammatory foods like turmeric, ginger, and omega-3-rich foods such as salmon and flaxseeds can help reduce chronic inflammation—a root cause of many diseases. Meal planning and preparing foods at home can make it easier to control ingredients and portion sizes, ensuring that every meal contributes positively to your health.

Physical Activity for Vitality Exercise is not just about weight management; it's crucial for maintaining cardiovascular health, strengthening muscles and bones, and enhancing mood and energy levels. Integrating regular physical activity into your schedule—whether it's yoga, walking, cycling, or strength training—ensures that your body's systems are balanced and functioning optimally. Even simple changes like taking the stairs instead of the elevator or short walking breaks during the workday can significantly boost your overall activity level.

Mindfulness and Mental Health Stress management is paramount in a holistic approach to health. Techniques such as meditation, deep breathing exercises, and mindfulness can greatly reduce stress levels and improve mental clarity and emotional stability. Allocating specific times for these practices, like meditating for a few minutes each morning or practicing deep breathing exercises during breaks, can help integrate these habits into daily life seamlessly.

Quality Sleep as a Healing Tool Quality sleep is critical for physical repair and mental health. Establishing a regular sleep schedule, creating a restful environment free from distractions, and avoiding stimulants like caffeine late in the day can enhance sleep quality. Natural aids such as lavender essential oil or chamomile tea before bedtime can also promote relaxation and help achieve deeper sleep cycles.

Community and Relationships Building and maintaining healthy relationships also contribute to overall well-being. Social interactions can reduce stress, improve mood, and provide emotional support. Engaging with community activities or group fitness classes can provide social and physical benefits simultaneously.

By weaving these natural healing practices into the fabric of daily life, you create a balanced and health-enhancing lifestyle that not only prevents disease but also enriches your quality of life. Each day offers opportunities to make choices that lead to a healthier, happier you.

Embracing the Full Spectrum of Holistic Healing

Dr. Barbara O'Neill's approach to holistic healing transcends conventional medical wisdom by emphasizing the interconnectedness of the human body with the mind and environment. Her methodology guides individuals to reclaim their health through natural, time-honored wisdom, focusing on the whole being rather than isolated symptoms.

Dr. Barbara champions a nourishing diet centered on organic, unprocessed foods, highlighting the importance of meals that are as vibrant and colorful as they are nutritious—each color providing different antioxidants and phytochemicals essential for combating diseases and enhancing vitality.

Her teachings extend into the ancient practice of herbal medicine, revealing how everyday herbs can significantly influence one's health. From the calming effects of chamomile to the digestive support of ginger, integrating herbal remedies into daily routines can prevent and address a plethora of health issues, strengthening the body's defenses and promoting recovery.

Another cornerstone of her philosophy is detoxification, a crucial aspect often overlooked in modern medicine. She offers practical advice on regular detox routines that cleanse the body's various systems, enhancing their functionality and thereby increasing overall well-being. Whether through periodic fasting, specialized diets, or the strategic use of supplements like milk thistle for liver health, her strategies are designed to purge toxins and renew the body.

Furthermore, Dr. Barbara places significant emphasis on mental health and emotional well-being, teaching that stress and emotional turmoil can lead to physical ailments. She introduces techniques such as mindfulness meditation, deep breathing exercises, and yoga—practices that not only reduce stress but also heighten awareness, leading to a more balanced and mindful approach to everyday living.

Dr. Barbara's holistic teachings encourage not just addressing specific ailments but fostering an environment where health can thrive. This includes creating a balanced lifestyle that aligns with natural rhythms and cycles, ensuring that sleep, exercise, and work-life balance are harmonized to support the body's natural healing abilities.

Through her holistic approach, you learn that every choice made is an opportunity to influence your health and that each day is a chance to live more harmoniously with nature's laws, leading to a healthier, happier existence.

The Philosophy of Whole-Body Wellness

Dr. Barbara's approach to health is revolutionary yet grounded in the simplicity of nature. She teaches that true health is more than the absence of disease; it's a vibrant state of energy and vitality. This can only be achieved by looking at the body as a whole—a complex system where everything is connected. Her philosophy underscores the importance of nurturing every aspect of oneself— physical, mental, spiritual, and emotional.

Physical Wellness Physical wellness, according to Dr. Barbara, is not just about avoiding illness but achieving optimal function and energy. This involves a balanced diet rich in whole, unprocessed foods that provide essential nutrients, vitamins, and minerals. Regular physical activity is also paramount. She advocates for exercise that suits an individual's lifestyle and preferences, from yoga and pilates to running and strength training, emphasizing that movement is essential for maintaining muscle mass, flexibility, and cardiovascular health.

Mental Wellness Mental wellness is equally critical in Dr. Barbara's holistic approach. She emphasizes the power of a positive mindset and the impact of thoughts on physical health. Techniques such as mindfulness, meditation, and mental exercises are encouraged to enhance cognitive function, reduce stress, and improve overall mental clarity. Dr. Barbara believes that mental health practices should be as routine as physical exercise, integrated seamlessly into daily life to maintain balance and reduce the risk of mental health disorders.

Spiritual Wellness Spiritual wellness involves connecting with something greater than oneself, which can provide a sense of purpose and fulfillment. This doesn't necessarily mean religious practices, although for some it might. It can also mean engaging in activities that bring joy and meaning, such as spending time in nature, practicing gratitude, or participating in community service. Dr. Barbara highlights that spiritual health can greatly influence emotional and physical well-being, providing resilience in the face of life's challenges.

Emotional Wellness Emotional wellness is about understanding and managing one's emotions.

Dr. Barbara teaches that emotional health can affect physical health, and vice versa. She advocates for practices that promote emotional balance, such as developing healthy relationships, expressing emotions through creative outlets, and practicing self-care. Techniques like journaling, therapy, and emotional release exercises are recommended to help individuals process and release emotional stress, contributing to overall well-being.

Interconnectedness and Balance Central to Dr. Barbara's philosophy is the interconnectedness of these wellness dimensions. She believes that neglecting any one aspect can lead to imbalances that manifest as physical or mental health issues. Therefore, her approach is holistic, aiming to harmonize the body, mind, and spirit. By nurturing each part of oneself, individuals can achieve a state of balance that supports a vibrant, healthy life.

Dr. Barbara's teachings encourage a proactive approach to health, where individuals take responsibility for their well-being through informed choices and consistent practices. This holistic view acknowledges that true health is dynamic and multifaceted, requiring attention to all aspects of life. Through her philosophy of whole-body wellness, Dr. Barbara provides a roadmap to not just live, but to thrive, in every sense of the word.

Diet: The Core of Vitality

One of Dr. Barbara's core tenets is that food is medicine. She advocates for a diet rich in whole, unprocessed foods that are as close to their natural state as possible. This approach emphasizes the profound impact that nutrition has on overall health and vitality.

Whole, Unprocessed Foods Dr. Barbara champions the consumption of whole, unprocessed foods, which retain their natural nutrients and are free from harmful additives. This includes fresh fruits and vegetables, whole grains, nuts, seeds, lean proteins, and healthy fats. By focusing on foods in their most natural form, you can ensure that you're receiving the maximum amount of vitamins, minerals, and antioxidants essential for maintaining optimal health.

Anti-Inflammatory Foods Integrating anti-inflammatory foods into your diet is a key aspect of Dr. Barbara's nutritional philosophy. Turmeric and ginger, for instance, are powerful anti-inflammatory agents that can help reduce chronic inflammation, a root cause of many diseases. These spices can be easily incorporated into daily meals, enhancing both flavor and health benefits.

Fermented Foods for Gut Health Dr. Barbara places significant emphasis on the importance of gut health, highlighting the benefits of fermented foods. Items like yogurt, kefir, sauerkraut, and kimchi are rich in probiotics, which are beneficial bacteria that help maintain a healthy gut flora. A balanced gut microbiome is crucial for efficient digestion, nutrient absorption, and a robust immune system. Regular consumption of fermented foods can support gut health, prevent digestive issues, and enhance overall well-being.

Detoxifying Foods Detoxification is another pillar of Dr. Barbara's dietary recommendations. She suggests incorporating foods that naturally detoxify the body, such as leafy greens, beets, garlic, and green tea. These foods help to cleanse the liver, kidneys, and colon, eliminating toxins and supporting the body's natural detox processes. Including these foods in your daily diet can enhance your body's ability to detoxify and rejuvenate at a cellular level.

Hydration and its Importance Adequate hydration is also a fundamental component of Dr. Barbara's dietary guidance. Drinking plenty of water is essential for maintaining bodily functions, aiding digestion, and flushing out toxins. She also recommends hydrating with natural beverages like herbal teas and infused waters, which can provide additional health benefits without added sugars or artificial ingredients.

Balanced and Varied Diet Dr. Barbara emphasizes the importance of a balanced and varied diet. This means consuming a wide range of foods to ensure that you're getting a diverse array of nutrients. A varied diet not only helps prevent nutrient deficiencies but also makes meals more enjoyable and satisfying. She encourages experimenting with different fruits, vegetables, grains, and proteins to keep your diet interesting and nutritionally comprehensive.

Mindful Eating Practices Mindful eating is another critical aspect of Dr. Barbara's dietary approach. She advocates for paying attention to what you eat, savoring each bite, and listening to your body's hunger and satiety cues. This practice helps prevent overeating, improves digestion, and fosters a healthier relationship with food. Mindful eating encourages you to appreciate the flavors and textures of your meals, making eating a more enjoyable and healthful experience.

By embracing these dietary principles, you can transform your eating habits and enhance your health significantly. Dr. Barbara's approach to nutrition is not just about feeding the body, but nourishing it deeply, promoting vitality, and supporting long-term health. Through her guidance, you learn that every meal is an opportunity to heal and energize, making food a cornerstone of a healthy, vibrant life.

Herbal Wisdom: Nature's Pharmacy

Herbs play a crucial role in Dr. Barbara's holistic health regimen, providing natural, potent remedies that support and enhance overall well-being. This approach taps into centuries-old traditions of using plants for their therapeutic properties, offering a natural alternative to synthetic medications.

Echinacea for Immune Support Echinacea is one of Dr. Barbara's top herb choices, renowned for its immune-boosting properties. Regular use of echinacea can help ward off colds and infections by stimulating the body's natural defenses. It can be taken as a tea, tincture, or supplement, especially during the cold and flu season, to enhance the immune response and reduce the severity and duration of illnesses.

Lavender for Relaxation and Sleep Lavender is celebrated for its calming effects, making it an excellent choice for promoting relaxation and improving sleep quality. Dr. Barbara often recommends using lavender in various forms, such as essential oils for aromatherapy, teas, or infused in bathwater. Its soothing aroma helps alleviate stress, anxiety, and insomnia, supporting mental and emotional well-being.

Garlic for Cardiovascular Health Garlic is another staple in Dr. Barbara's herbal repertoire, known for its cardiovascular benefits. It helps lower blood pressure, reduce cholesterol levels, and improve overall heart health. Garlic can be easily incorporated into the diet through cooking, or taken as a supplement. Its natural antibiotic and antiviral properties also make it a valuable tool for boosting immunity.

Creating Herbal Tinctures Dr. Barbara emphasizes the effectiveness of herbal tinctures, which are concentrated liquid extracts of herbs. Tinctures are easy to make at home by soaking herbs in alcohol or glycerin for several weeks. This method extracts the active compounds, creating a potent remedy that can be used for various ailments. For example, an echinacea tincture can be taken at the first sign of a cold to boost immunity.

Herbal Teas for Daily Wellness Herbal teas are a simple and enjoyable way to incorporate the benefits of herbs into daily life. Dr. Barbara suggests making teas from herbs like chamomile for relaxation, peppermint for digestive support, and ginger for anti-inflammatory effects. These teas can be consumed regularly to maintain health and prevent common issues.

Salves and Topical Applications Herbal salves and ointments are excellent for treating skin conditions, wounds, and muscle pain. Dr. Barbara recommends creating salves using herbs like calendula for its healing and anti-inflammatory properties, and comfrey for promoting tissue repair. These can be applied directly to the skin to soothe and heal.

Daily Herbal Supplements Integrating herbs into daily supplements can significantly enhance long-term wellness. Herbs such as turmeric for its anti-inflammatory properties, milk thistle for liver support, and ashwagandha for stress reduction can be taken in capsule form to provide consistent health benefits. Dr. Barbara advises choosing high-quality supplements and consulting with a healthcare provider to tailor them to individual health needs.

Personalizing Herbal Use One of Dr. Barbara's key teachings is the importance of personalizing herbal use to suit individual health conditions and goals. She encourages learning about the specific benefits and uses of various herbs and experimenting with different combinations to find what works best. This personalized approach ensures that herbal remedies are effective and aligned with one's unique health profile.

Sustainable and Ethical Herbal Practices Dr. Barbara also stresses the importance of sustainable and ethical practices in herbal medicine. This includes sourcing herbs responsibly, growing your own when possible, and respecting traditional knowledge and practices. Ethical herbalism not only supports personal health but also the health of the environment and communities.

Embracing the wisdom of nature's pharmacy allows you to harness the healing power of plants, creating a foundation for long-term wellness. Through her herbal teachings, Dr. Barbara empowers you to take charge of your health in a natural, sustainable way, integrating the profound benefits of herbs into your everyday life.

The Power of Detoxification

Detoxification is a cornerstone of Dr. Barbara's health philosophy, vital for maintaining a body free from the accumulation of harmful substances. This practice supports the liver, kidneys, and colon, helping to remove toxins and enhance the body's natural healing processes.

Liver Cleansing The liver is a central organ in detoxification, processing and eliminating toxins from the body. Dr. Barbara recommends several strategies to support liver health. Consuming liver-friendly foods such as beets, dandelion greens, and milk thistle can significantly enhance liver function. Milk thistle, in particular, contains silymarin, a compound known for its liver-protective properties. Incorporating these foods into your diet can promote liver regeneration and improve detoxification efficiency.

Kidney Support The kidneys filter waste and excess substances from the blood, excreting them through urine. Dr. Barbara advocates for staying well-hydrated to support kidney function, emphasizing the importance of drinking plenty of water and herbal teas. Herbs like nettle and parsley can act as natural diuretics, helping to flush out toxins. Reducing sodium intake and consuming potassium-rich foods like bananas and sweet potatoes can also aid kidney health.

Colon Cleansing Maintaining a healthy colon is crucial for effective detoxification. Dr. Barbara suggests incorporating high-fiber foods such as fruits, vegetables, whole grains, and legumes into your diet to promote regular bowel movements and prevent the buildup of waste in the colon. She also recommends periodic colon cleanses using natural methods like water or herbal colon cleansing formulas to remove accumulated toxins.

Juicing for Detox Juicing is a powerful detoxification tool, providing a concentrated source of vitamins, minerals, and antioxidants. Dr. Barbara recommends juicing fresh, organic fruits and vegetables to create nutrient-dense beverages that support the body's detox processes. Ingredients like leafy greens, carrots, apples, and ginger are particularly effective. Juicing allows for the quick absorption of nutrients while giving the digestive system a rest.

Fasting Fasting is another detoxification method endorsed by Dr. Barbara, offering a break for the digestive system and allowing the body to focus on healing and repair. Intermittent fasting, where eating is restricted to a specific window of time each day, can be a practical and manageable approach. Longer fasting periods, such as 24-hour or multi-day fasts, can also be beneficial but should be undertaken with caution and possibly under medical supervision.

Castor Oil Packs Castor oil packs are a unique detoxification technique promoted by Dr. Barbara. When applied to the skin over the liver or abdomen, castor oil packs can improve circulation, reduce inflammation, and promote the elimination of toxins. To make a castor oil pack, soak a piece of flannel in castor oil, place it on the desired area, cover with plastic wrap, and apply heat using a heating pad. Leave the pack on for 30-60 minutes to allow the oil to penetrate deeply and stimulate detoxification.

Herbal Detox Teas Herbal teas are an effective and gentle way to support detoxification. Dr. Barbara recommends teas made from herbs such as dandelion root, burdock root, and green tea, which have natural detoxifying properties. These teas can help cleanse the liver, kidneys, and digestive tract, promoting overall detoxification and health.

Sweat Therapy Sweating is a natural way to eliminate toxins through the skin. Dr. Barbara suggests incorporating regular physical activity, sauna sessions, or hot baths to induce sweating and support the detoxification process. These practices can help clear out toxins and improve circulation, enhancing the body's overall detox capacity.

Balanced Lifestyle Finally, Dr. Barbara emphasizes the importance of a balanced lifestyle in maintaining effective detoxification. This includes managing stress, getting adequate sleep, and avoiding exposure to environmental toxins. Practices such as yoga, meditation, and spending time in nature can support overall well-being and enhance the body's ability to detoxify.

Embracing Dr. Barbara's detoxification protocols can lead to significant improvements in health and vitality. By regularly cleansing the liver, kidneys, and colon, and incorporating natural detox methods into your lifestyle, you can support your body's innate healing abilities and achieve a state of optimal health.

Stress Management and Emotional Balance

Understanding and managing stress is vital for holistic health. Dr. Barbara emphasizes the destructive impact of stress on physical health, highlighting the need for effective techniques to cope with and thrive despite life's challenges.

The Impact of Stress on Health Stress triggers a cascade of physiological responses that can have detrimental effects on the body. Chronic stress can lead to high blood pressure, weakened immune function, digestive issues, and mental health disorders such as anxiety and depression. Dr. Barbara underscores that managing stress is not just about feeling better emotionally but also about preserving and enhancing physical health.

Deep Breathing Techniques Deep breathing is one of the simplest yet most effective ways to reduce stress. Dr. Barbara teaches that deep, diaphragmatic breathing can activate the body's relaxation response, reducing heart rate and blood pressure. Practicing deep breathing exercises, such as the 4-7-8 technique (inhale for 4 seconds, hold for 7 seconds, exhale for 8 seconds), can be done anywhere and at any time, providing immediate stress relief.

Yoga for Mind and Body Yoga combines physical postures, breathing exercises, and meditation to promote relaxation and well-being. Dr. Barbara advocates for regular yoga practice to enhance flexibility, strength, and mental clarity. The mindful movements and deep breathing associated with yoga help release physical tension and calm the mind, making it an excellent practice for reducing stress and promoting emotional balance. Incorporating yoga into daily routines, even for just a few minutes a day, can yield significant benefits.

Mindfulness Meditation Mindfulness meditation involves focusing on the present moment and observing thoughts and feelings without judgment. This practice helps reduce stress by breaking the cycle of negative thinking and promoting a sense of calm and clarity. Dr. Barbara recommends starting with short sessions of mindfulness meditation, gradually increasing the duration as you become more comfortable with the practice. Techniques such as body scan meditation, where you focus on different parts of the body and release tension, can be particularly effective.

Gratitude Practices Practicing gratitude can shift focus from stressors to positive aspects of life, fostering emotional balance and resilience. Dr. Barbara suggests keeping a gratitude journal, where you regularly write down things you are thankful for. This practice can help reframe your perspective, making it easier to manage stress and cultivate a more positive outlook.

Physical Activity Regular physical activity is a powerful stress reliever. Exercise releases endorphins, the body's natural mood enhancers, and helps reduce levels of the stress hormone cortisol. Dr. Barbara encourages incorporating various forms of exercise, such as walking, running, dancing, or swimming, into your routine. Finding activities that you enjoy can make exercise a pleasurable and sustainable way to manage stress.

Healthy Sleep Habits Quality sleep is essential for emotional balance and stress management. Dr. Barbara highlights the importance of establishing a regular sleep schedule, creating a restful environment, and avoiding stimulants like caffeine before bedtime. Practices such as reading, taking a warm bath, or practicing gentle stretches before bed can promote relaxation and improve sleep quality.

Balanced Lifestyle A balanced lifestyle that includes adequate rest, nutrition, and leisure activities is crucial for managing stress. Dr. Barbara advocates for a holistic approach to health, where all aspects of life are harmonized to support well-being. This includes setting boundaries, prioritizing self-care, and making time for activities that bring joy and relaxation.

Social Connections Maintaining strong social connections is vital for emotional health. Dr. Barbara emphasizes the importance of nurturing relationships with family, friends, and community. Engaging in social activities, seeking support from loved ones, and participating in group activities can provide a sense of belonging and reduce feelings of isolation and stress.

Creative Outlets Engaging in creative activities such as painting, writing, music, or gardening can be therapeutic and help manage stress. Dr. Barbara encourages exploring different creative outlets to find what resonates with you. These activities can provide a sense of accomplishment, improve mood, and offer a break from daily stressors.

By integrating these stress management techniques into your daily routine, you can significantly reduce stress levels and promote emotional balance. Dr. Barbara's holistic approach to stress management not only helps alleviate the immediate effects of stress but also builds long-term resilience, enabling you to navigate life's challenges with greater ease and well-being.

Integrative Practices: Bringing It All Together

Integrative practices are the culmination of Dr. Barbara's teachings, synthesizing nutrition, herbal wisdom, detoxification, and stress management into a cohesive and personalized health plan. This approach encourages a proactive stance towards health, emphasizing the importance of preventive measures alongside reactive treatments.

Creating a Personalized Health Plan Dr. Barbara advocates for a tailored approach to health, recognizing that each individual's needs are unique. Start by assessing your current lifestyle, diet, and health status. Identify areas that need improvement and set realistic goals. Incorporate whole, unprocessed foods into your diet, ensuring a balance of macronutrients and a variety of fruits and vegetables. Regularly include detoxifying foods and practices to support liver, kidney, and colon health.

Daily Routine Integration To achieve consistency, integrate health practices into your daily routine. Begin the day with mindfulness meditation or deep breathing exercises to set a positive tone. Include physical activity that you enjoy, whether it's a morning jog, yoga session, or evening walk. Plan meals ahead to ensure they are balanced and nutrient-dense, making use of herbs and spices that support overall health.

Proactive Health Measures Adopting a proactive approach involves regular health check-ups, staying informed about your body's needs, and making adjustments as necessary. Utilize herbal tinctures and teas as daily supplements to boost immunity, support digestion, and enhance mental clarity. Engage in periodic detoxification routines, such as juicing or fasting, to cleanse your system and rejuvenate your body.

Stress Management Techniques Incorporate stress management techniques throughout your day. Practice gratitude journaling in the morning, take short breaks to practice deep breathing or stretch, and engage in activities that promote relaxation and joy. Ensure you maintain strong social connections and seek support when needed.

Holistic Lifestyle Choices Making holistic choices involves more than just diet and exercise. It's about creating an environment that supports your well-being. Ensure your living space is clean and free of toxins, use natural products, and spend time in nature to reconnect with its healing energies. Balance work and leisure, and prioritize sleep and rest to allow your body to recover and regenerate.

Real-World Transformations The power of Dr. Barbara's holistic health methods is evidenced by countless individuals who have transformed their lives. Take inspiration from stories of people who have overcome chronic illnesses, improved their mental health, and achieved a higher quality of life through her teachings. These real-world examples demonstrate the profound impact of embracing a holistic approach to health.

Continuous Learning and Adaptation Health is a dynamic journey that requires continuous learning and adaptation. Stay curious and informed about new health practices and scientific discoveries. Dr. Barbara encourages lifelong learning and being open to trying new methods that may benefit your health. Regularly review and adjust your health plan to ensure it remains effective and aligned with your goals.

By bringing together all aspects of Dr. Barbara's teachings, you can create a comprehensive and personalized health plan that promotes lasting wellness. This integrative approach not only addresses immediate health concerns but also builds a strong foundation for a healthy future, demonstrating the true power of holistic healing.

CONCLUSION
EMBRACING A LIFETIME OF HOLISTIC HEALTH

As we reach the end of this journey through Dr. Barbara O'Neill's teachings, it's clear that true health and vitality stem from a holistic approach that nurtures every aspect of our being. The wisdom and practices shared in this book offer a roadmap to a healthier, more balanced life, grounded in the principles of natural healing, preventive care, and proactive wellness.

Embracing the holistic health philosophy means recognizing the interconnectedness of our physical, mental, emotional, and spiritual selves. It involves making mindful choices every day that support our overall well-being, from the foods we eat to the thoughts we think, the activities we engage in, and the relationships we nurture.

Dr. Barbara's approach to nutrition, which emphasizes whole, unprocessed foods and the power of herbs, provides a solid foundation for physical health. By integrating detoxification practices, we can regularly cleanse our bodies, removing toxins and rejuvenating our systems. Stress management techniques and emotional balance strategies help us maintain mental clarity and emotional stability, essential components of holistic wellness.

The journey doesn't end here. The principles and practices outlined in this book are not just temporary fixes but lifelong habits that can transform your health. As you continue to explore and integrate these teachings into your life, remember to listen to your body, stay informed, and adapt your health plan as needed. Health is a dynamic, ever-evolving journey, and staying proactive and engaged is key to sustaining long-term wellness.

Reflect on the inspiring stories of individuals who have transformed their lives through Dr. Barbara's methods. Let their experiences motivate you to take charge of your health, embrace holistic practices, and trust in the natural wisdom of your body. You have the tools, knowledge, and guidance to create a vibrant, healthy life—one that is rich in energy, balance, and joy.

As you move forward, keep in mind the essence of Dr. Barbara's teachings: true health is more than the absence of disease; it is a state of complete physical, mental, and emotional well-being. By nurturing every aspect of yourself and making informed, mindful choices, you can achieve and maintain this state of holistic health.

Thank you for embarking on this journey towards a healthier, more fulfilling life. May the wisdom and practices shared in this book empower you to live each day with vitality, purpose, and harmony. Here's to a lifetime of holistic health and well-being.

  Dr. Barbara's Natural Healing Secrets